DUMBBELL TRAINING

Allen Hedrick

HUMAN KINETICS

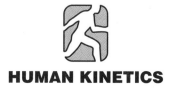

Library of Congress Cataloging-in-Publication Data

Hedrick, Allen.
 Dumbbell training / Allen Hedrick.
    pages cm
 Includes bibliographical references.
 1. Dumbbells. 2. Physical fitness. I. Title.
 GV547.4.H43 2014
 613.7'13--dc23

                              2013038726

ISBN-10: 1-4504-4458-X (print)
ISBN-13: 978-1-4504-4458-3 (print)

The web addresses cited in this text were current as of September 2013, unless otherwise noted.

Acquisitions Editor: Justin Klug; **Developmental Editor:** Anne Hall; **Assistant Editor:** Tyler M. Wolpert; **Copyeditor:** Annette Pierce; **Permissions Manager:** Martha Gullo; **Graphic Designer:** Joe Buck; **Cover Designer:** Keith Blomberg; **Photograph (cover):** Neil Bernstein; **Photographs (interior):** © Human Kinetics, unless otherwise noted. Permission to reprint the photo on p. xi granted under the terms of the GNU Free Documentation License. A copy of this license is available at http://commons.wikimedia.org/wiki/Commons:GNU_ Free_Documentation_License_1.2 [December 17, 2013]; **Photo Asset Manager:** Laura Fitch; **Visual Production Assistant:** Joyce Brumfield; **Photo Production Manager:** Jason Allen; **Art Manager:** Kelly Hendren; **Associate Art Manager:** Alan L. Wilborn; **Illustrations:** © Human Kinetics; **Printer:** Versa Press

We thank the Pack Strength & Conditioning Facility on the Campus of Colorado State University Pueblo for assistance in providing the location for the photo shoot for this book.

Human Kinetics
Website: www.HumanKinetics.com

United States: Human Kinetics
P.O. Box 5076
Champaign, IL 61825-5076
800-747-4457
e-mail: humank@hkusa.com

Canada: Human Kinetics
475 Devonshire Road Unit 100
Windsor, ON N8Y 2L5
800-465-7301 (in Canada only)
e-mail: info@hkcanada.com

Europe: Human Kinetics
107 Bradford Road
Stanningley
Leeds LS28 6AT, United Kingdom
+44 (0) 113 255 5665
e-mail: hk@hkeurope.com

Australia: Human Kinetics
57A Price Avenue
Lower Mitcham, South Australia 5062
08 8372 0999
e-mail: info@hkaustralia.com

New Zealand: Human Kinetics
P.O. Box 80
Torrens Park, South Australia 5062
0800 222 062
e-mail: info@hknewzealand.com

E5878

Contents

Exercise Finder

Exercise	Primary muscles worked	Other muscles worked	Single joint or multijoint	Page #
Chapter 4: Upper-Body				
SHOULDERS				
Front Raise	Anterior Deltoid	Pectoralis Major, Lateral Deltoid, Middle and Lower Trapezius	Single	42
Lateral Raise	Lateral Deltoid	Anterior Deltoid, Supraspinatus, Middle and Lower Trapezius, Serratus Anterior	Single	43
Shoulder Press	Anterior Deltoid	Lateral Deltoid, Supraspinatus, Triceps, Middle and Lower Trapezius, Serratus Anterior, Pectoralis Major	Multijoint	44
Alternating Shoulder Press	Anterior Deltoid	Lateral Deltoid, Supraspinatus, Triceps, Middle and Lower Trapezius, Serratus Anterior, Pectoralis Major	Multijoint	45
One-Arm Shoulder Press	Anterior Deltoid	Lateral Deltoid, Supraspinatus, Triceps, Middle and Lower Trapezius, Serratus Anterior, Pectoralis Major	Multijoint	46
Upright Row	Lateral Deltoid	Anterior Deltoid, Supraspinatus, Brachialis. Brachioradialis, Middle and Lower Trapezius, Serratus Anterior, Infraspinatus	Multijoint	47

Exercise	Primary muscles worked	Other muscles worked	Single joint or multijoint	Page #
CHEST				
Pullover	Pectoralis Major	Latissimus Dorsi, Teres Major, Triceps Posterior Deltoid, Pectoralis Minor, Rhomboids, Levator Scapulae	Single	48
Fly	Pectoralis Major	Anterior Deltoid, Biceps Brachii	Single	49
Incline Fly	Pectoralis Major	Anterior Deltoid, Biceps Brachii	Single	50
Decline Fly	Pectoralis Major	Anterior Deltoid, Biceps Brachii	Single	51
Incline Press	Pectoralis Major	Anterior Deltoid, Triceps	Multijoint	52
Alternating Incline Press	Pectoralis Major	Anterior Deltoid, Triceps	Multijoint	53
One-Arm Incline Press	Pectoralis Major	Anterior Deltoid, Triceps	Multijoint	54
Decline Press	Pectoralis Major	Anterior Deltoid, Triceps	Multijoint	55
Alternating Decline Press	Pectoralis Major	Anterior Deltoid, Triceps	Multijoint	56
One-Arm Decline Press	Pectoralis Major	Anterior Deltoid, Triceps	Multijoint	57
Bench Press	Pectoralis Major	Anterior Deltoid, Triceps	Multijoint	58
Alternating Bench Press	Pectoralis Major	Anterior Deltoid, Triceps	Multijoint	59
One-Arm Bench Press	Pectoralis Major	Anterior Deltoid, Triceps	Multijoint	60
UPPER BACK				
Row	Latissimus Dorsi	Trapezius, Rhomboids, Biceps Brachii, Erector Spinae	Multijoint	61
BICEPS				
Curl	Biceps Brachii,	Brachialis, Brachioradialis	Single	62
Hammer Curl	Brachioradialis, Biceps Brachii	Anterior Deltoid, Trapezius, Levator Scapulae	Single	63
Reverse Curl	Brachioradialis, Biceps Brachii	Anterior Deltoid, Trapezius, Levator Scapulae	Single	64

(continued)

Exercise	Primary muscles worked	Other muscles worked	Single joint or multijoint	Page #
Straight-Leg Deadlift	Hamstrings	Erector Spinae, Gluteus Maximus, Adductor Magnus	Multijoint	83
Calf Raise	Gastrocnemius	Soleus	Single	84
Step-Up	Quadriceps	Gluteus Maximus, Adductor Magnus, Soleus, Gastrocnemius	Multijoint	85
Chapter 6: Core				
ABDOMINALS				
Crunch	Rectus Abdominis	Obliques	Multijoint	88
Decline Crunch	Rectus Abdominis	Obliques	Multijoint	89
Twisting Crunch	Obliques	Rectus Abdominis, Psoas Major	Multijoint	90
Decline Twisting Crunch	Obliques	Rectus Abdominis, Psoas Major	Multijoint	91
Toe Touch	Rectus Abdominis	Obliques	Multijoint	92
Alternating Toe Touch	Rectus Abdominis	Obliques	Multijoint	93
V-Up	Rectus Abdominis	Iliopsoas, Tensor Fasciae Latae, Pectineus, Sartorius, Rectus Femoris, Adductor Longus, Adductor Brevis, Obliques	Multijoint	94
Alternating V-Up	Rectus Abdominis	Iliopsoas, Tensor Fasciae Latae, Pectineus, Sartorius, Rectus Femoris, Adductor Longus, Adductor Brevis, Obliques	Multijoint	95
Press Crunch	Rectus Abdominis	Obliques	Multijoint	96
Decline Press Crunch	Rectus Abdominis	Obliques	Multijoint	97
Alternating Press Crunch	Rectus Abdominis	Obliques	Multijoint	98
Decline Alternating Press Crunch	Rectus Abdominis	Obliques	Multijoint	99
LOWER BACK				
Back Extension	Erector Spinae	Gluteus Maximus, Hamstrings, Adductor Magnus	Multijoint	100
Twisting Back Extension	Erector Spinae	Gluteus Maximus, Hamstrings, Adductor Magnus	Multijoint	102

(continued)

Exercise	Primary muscles worked	Other muscles worked	Single joint or multijoint	Page #
Chapter 7: Total-Body				
Push Press	Quadriceps, Gastrocnemius, Gluteus Maximus, Hamstrings	Deltoids, Triceps, Rectus Abdominis, Erector Spinae,	Multijoint	106
Alternating Push Press	Quadriceps, Gastrocnemius, Gluteus Maximus, Hamstrings	Deltoids, Triceps, Rectus Abdominis, Erector Spinae	Multijoint	107
One-Arm Push Press	Quadriceps, Gastrocnemius, Gluteus Maximus, Hamstrings	Deltoids, Triceps, Rectus Abdominis, Erector Spinae	Multijoint	108
Power Jerk	Quadriceps, Gastrocnemius, Gluteus Maximus, Hamstrings	Deltoids, Triceps, Rectus Abdominis, Erector Spinae	Multijoint	109
Alternating Power Jerk	Quadriceps, Gastrocnemius, Gluteus Maximus, Hamstrings	Deltoids, Triceps, Rectus Abdominis, Erector Spinae	Multijoint	110
One-Arm Power Jerk	Quadriceps, Gastrocnemius, Gluteus Maximus, Hamstrings	Deltoids, Triceps, Rectus Abdominis, Erector Spinae	Multijoint	111
Split Alternating-Feet Jerk	Quadriceps, Gastrocnemius, Gluteus Maximus, Hamstrings	Deltoids, Triceps, Rectus Abdominis, Erector Spinae	Multijoint	112
Split Alternating-Feet Alternating-Arm Jerk	Quadriceps, Gastrocnemius, Gluteus Maximus, Hamstrings	Deltoids, Triceps, Rectus Abdominis, Erector Spinae	Multijoint	114
Split Alternating-Feet One-Arm Jerk	Quadriceps, Gastrocnemius, Gluteus Maximus, Hamstrings	Deltoids, Triceps, Rectus Abdominis, Erector Spinae	Multijoint	116
Hang Power Clean	Quadriceps, Gastrocnemius, Gluteus Maximus, Hamstrings	Trapezius, Latissimus Dorsi, Biceps Brachii, Rectus Abdominis, Erector Spinae, Deltoids, Triceps	Multijoint	118
Alternating Power Clean	Quadriceps, Gastrocnemius, Gluteus Maximus, Hamstrings	Trapezius, Latissimus Dorsi, Biceps Brachii, Rectus Abdominis, Erector Spinae, Deltoids, Triceps	Multijoint	120

Exercise	Primary muscles worked	Other muscles worked	Single joint or multijoint	Page #
One-Arm Power Clean	Quadriceps, Gastrocnemius, Gluteus Maximus, Hamstrings	Trapezius, Latissimus Dorsi, Biceps Brachii, Rectus Abdominis, Erector Spinae, Deltoids, Triceps	Multijoint	122
Hang Clean	Quadriceps, Gastrocnemius, Gluteus Maximus, Hamstrings	Trapezius, Latissimus Dorsi, Biceps Brachii, Rectus Abdominis, Erector Spinae, Deltoids, Triceps	Multijoint	124
Alternating Hang Clean	Quadriceps, Gastrocnemius, Gluteus Maximus, Hamstrings	Trapezius, Latissimus Dorsi, Biceps Brachii, Rectus Abdominis, Erector Spinae, Deltoids, Triceps	Multijoint	126
One-Arm Hang Clean	Quadriceps, Gastrocnemius, Gluteus Maximus, Hamstrings	Trapezius, Latissimus Dorsi, Biceps Brachii, Rectus Abdominis, Erector Spinae, Deltoids, Triceps	Multijoint	128
Power Snatch	Quadriceps, Gastrocnemius, Gluteus Maximus, Hamstrings	Trapezius, Latissimus Dorsi, Rectus Abdominis, Erector Spinae, Deltoids, Triceps	Multijoint	130
Alternating Power Snatch	Quadriceps, Gastrocnemius, Gluteus Maximus, Hamstrings	Trapezius, Latissimus Dorsi, Biceps Brachii, Rectus Abdominis, Erector Spinae, Deltoids, Triceps	Multijoint	132
One-Arm Power Snatch	Quadriceps, Gastrocnemius, Gluteus Maximus, Hamstrings	Trapezius, Latissimus Dorsi, Rectus Abdominis, Erector Spinae, Deltoids, Triceps	Multijoint	134
Split Alternating-Feet Snatch	Quadriceps, Gastrocnemius, Gluteus Maximus, Hamstrings	Trapezius, Latissimus Dorsi, Rectus Abdominis, Erector Spinae, Deltoids, Triceps	Multijoint	136
Split Alternating-Feet Alternating-Arm Snatch	Quadriceps, Gastrocnemius, Gluteus Maximus, Hamstrings	Trapezius, Latissimus Dorsi, Rectus Abdominis, Erector Spinae, Deltoids, Triceps	Multijoint	138
One-Arm Split Alternating-Feet Snatch	Quadriceps, Gastrocnemius, Gluteus Maximus, Hamstrings	Trapezius, Latissimus Dorsi, Rectus Abdominis, Erector Spinae, Deltoids, Triceps	Multijoint	140

Introduction

The use of dumbbells as a resistance training modality has a long history. After a brief review of that history, we will look at the types of dumbbells and their uses and the equipment needed to perform the exercises in this book.

The earliest predecessors of the dumbbell were halteres (shown in figure 1), used in ancient Greece similarly to how we use dumbbells today. Halteres were made of stone or metal and weighed between two and nine kilograms (4.4-19.8 lbs). The halteres were shaped or carved to include a handle that made it easier to grip the implement. Although the ancient Egyptians, Chinese, Indians, and many other people practiced resistance training, credit traditionally has been given to the Greeks for producing the predecessor of modern weight training equipment. In addition to using halteres for resistance training, the ancient Greeks also used them when performing their version of the long jump. The athletes held an implement in each hand in an attempt to increase the distance of their jumps. Interestingly, some ancient texts also use the term halteres to describe the weapon used by David to slay Goliath (Todd 2003).

Indian clubs, similar in form to dumbbells, were used in India for more than a thousand years. Indian clubs were also popular in the late 19th and early 20th centuries in Europe, the British Commonwealth, and the United

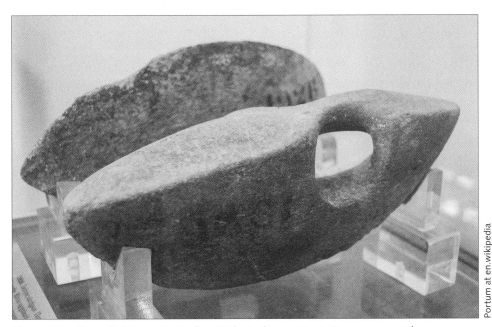

Portum at en.wikipedia

Figure 1   Stone halteres, typically attributed to ancient Greece, were the predecessor to modern strength equipment.

States. Because the implement is shaped like a club, it became known as an Indian club. The bowling-pin shaped wooden club came in various sizes and weights. During training, athletes swung the Indian clubs in specific patterns. Clubs ranged from a few pounds (about 1 kg) each, up to special clubs that weighed as much as 50 pounds (22.6 kg). Indian clubs were normally used in pairs during training in carefully choreographed routines in which a group of exercisers, led by an instructor, swung the clubs in unison. The routines varied based on the ability of the athletes and the weight of the clubs.

The term dumbbells may have originated in Tudor England and referred to equipment simulating the action of ringing a church bell used by people learning the technique and building the strength required for English bell ringing. The clapper in the bell was tied back so that no sound was produced. As a result, the equipment was referred to as dumb-bells. When athletes started to make their own equipment for strength training, they kept the name dumbbell, even though the shape of the equipment had changed. In the early 17th century, dumbbells were manufactured that began to resemble the dumbbell we are familiar with today.

The three primary types of dumbbells are adjustable, fixed, and selectorized. Adjustable dumbbells consist of a metal handle and weight plates. Often the center of the handle is engraved to create a knurling effect to improve grip. Weight plates slide onto the ends of the handle and are secured with clips or collars. The advantage of this system is that it requires only two handles and the required weight plates to create two evenly loaded dumbbells, producing a variety of weights.

The disadvantage of this system is that nearly every time you perform a different exercise (e.g., dumbbell lateral raises, dumbbell squats) the weight needs to be changed. Further, especially for athletes with an extensive training background, a large range of loading capabilities will be required as strength increases and it becomes necessary to increase the training load.

Fixed-weight dumbbells are often made of cast iron, either molded in the shape of a dumbbell or consisting of individual weight plates permanently attached to a handle. Sometimes the weight plates are coated with rubber or neoprene, which offers padding and protects the floor. A less expensive (and less durable) type of fixed-weight dumbbell is made of concrete and coated with rubber.

The primary advantage of fixed-weight dumbbells is that you do not have to change the load on the dumbbell when you start the next exercise. Instead, you simply grab the dumbbells of the desired weight and you are ready to go. The disadvantage of fixed-weight dumbbells, in comparison to adjustable dumbbells, is that you need many dumbbells to cover the weight range required to perform a variety of exercises. A relatively new model of dumbbell, at least in comparison to the other types, is the selectorized dumbbell. Athletes select the weight on the dumbbell by turning a dial or moving a selector pin to a specific weight rather than changing weight plates. A selectorized dumbbell is a set of weights sitting in a dumbbell holder. The dumbbell handle sits inside a series of weighted plates. By turning a knob or sliding a pin into the dumbbell holder the desired weight can be selected. Only the selected weight is attached to the handle when the handle is removed from the dumbbell holder. Selectorized dumbbells have a similar advantage to adjustable dumbbells in that only two dumbbells are required rather than a pair of dumbbells of each weight. A disadvantage of selectorized dumbbells is that every time you want to adjust the weight, you need to add or remove weights. This is not a major issue, but it does add to training time.

Besides the dumbbells themselves, not a lot of additional equipment is required for most dumbbell exercises. One piece of equipment that is helpful is an exercise bench that can adjust from flat to both incline and decline. This allows you to perform, for example, dumbbell bench presses, dumbbell incline presses, and dumbbell decline presses. You can use the same bench when performing one-leg squats and dumbbell rows. An attachment that anchors your legs when the bench is declined is useful when performing decline abdominal exercises.

During some exercises, such as bench press and incline press, it is difficult to place the dumbbells gently on the floor after performing a heavy set. Because it is important that setting down the dumbbells does not damage the floor, another useful piece of equipment is a four-by-eight-foot (1.2-by-2.4-cm) rubber mat or other product such as three-quarter-inch (2 cm) plywood. It is also recommended that you perform the total-body exercises on a mat or sheet of plywood to protect the floor. These explosive total-body movements can be fatiguing, which can make it difficult to place the dumbbells gently on the floor at the completion of the set.

Other than the dumbbells, an adjustable bench, and a rubber mat or piece of plywood to protect the floor, no other equipment is required to perform the dumbbell exercises in this book. Chapters 1-3 discuss the benefits of training with dumbbells and how to design an appropriate plan using dumbbells or incorporate them into your current training plan.

After reviewing the correct technique for an extensive list of exercises performed with dumbbells in chapters 4-7, chapters 8 and 9 discuss how to increase muscle size and power. Moving on, example workouts for a variety of sports are found in chapters 10-12. Chapter 10 is focused on training for power sports (e.g., throwers in track, basketball, volleyball). Next, chapter 11 looks at training for speed sports (e.g., track sprinter, swim sprinter, cyclist sprinter). Finally, chapter 12 is aimed at training for agility and balance sports (e.g., wrestling, soccer, ice hockey, downhill skiing). While obviously every sport cannot be covered in this book, the example workouts provide the information needed to allow you to design an effective workout for whatever sport you may participate in.

Key to Muscles

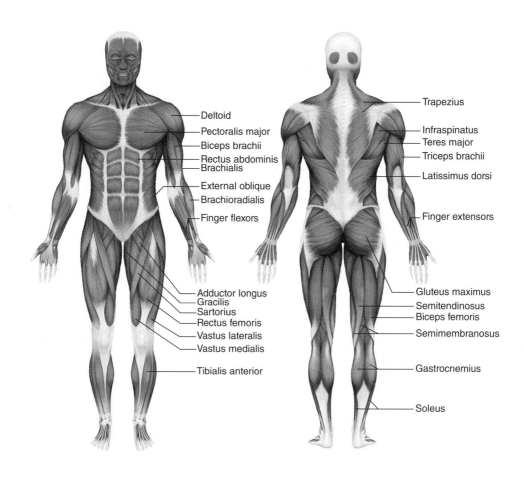

Deltoid
Pectoralis major
Biceps brachii
Rectus abdominis
Brachialis
External oblique
Brachioradialis
Finger flexors

Adductor longus
Gracilis
Sartorius
Rectus femoris
Vastus lateralis
Vastus medialis
Tibialis anterior

Trapezius
Infraspinatus
Teres major
Triceps brachii
Latissimus dorsi

Finger extensors

Gluteus maximus
Semitendinosus
Biceps femoris
Semimembranosus

Gastrocnemius

Soleus

PART I

TRAINING WITH DUMBBELLS

Training with dumbbells can be a lot of hard work. And most people, before engaging in rigorous exercise, want to know what the benefits will be before agreeing to participate in a challenging training program. The reality is that including dumbbells in your training program reaps significant benefits.

Some of the benefits are practical: The equipment is low cost and doesn't take up much space. And some of the benefits are physiological. Research has shown that activation of the pectoral muscles during a dumbbell bench press is similar to activation when performing the same exercise with a barbell. Further, activation of the core muscles is greater when training with dumbbells than when training with a barbell because of the need to control two separate implements.

It may seem that writing a resistance training program emphasizing dumbbell training would be difficult, but the process is quite easy. The vast majority of barbell exercises, or machine exercises for that matter, can be performed with dumbbells. For example, turning a barbell squat into a dumbbell squat is primarily a matter of using different equipment. Converting a machine leg press requires finding a dumbbell exercise that trains the same muscle groups. In this case, it's dumbbell squats. Similarly, barbell bent rows or machine seated rows become dumbbell rows.

Let's take a more thorough look at those benefits so you have a greater understanding of what training with dumbbells can do for you. The more you know and understand about these potential benefits, the better you will be able to create an effective training program.

Benefits of Training With Dumbbells

Training with dumbbells provides a variety of advantages. Some of the advantages are practical and some are physiological, but without a doubt, dumbbells will be a good addition to your training program.

PRACTICAL ADVANTAGES OF DUMBBELLS

Let's start by looking at the practical advantages. One significant benefit of training with dumbbells is their relative low cost and adaptability in comparison with other modes of training. Most exercise machines are expensive and typically can be used to perform only one exercise.

Dumbbells, on the other hand, provide a huge range of exercises. And nearly every barbell exercise you can think of can also be performed with dumbbells. But that is not the end of the list. Add all the exercise variations that are possible with dumbbells that are not possible with barbells (e.g., single-arm and alternating-arm exercises) and you quickly see that the number of potential dumbbell exercises is quite large.

Another benefit of dumbbell training over machine training is that most machines do not lend themselves well to explosive training, the importance of which is discussed in chapter 7. Dumbbells are well suited to explosive training, which is the focus of most of the dumbbell exercises my athletes perform.

While barbells and weight plates are less expensive than exercise machines, they cost more than dumbbells. Further, many exercises performed with barbells require specialized equipment, such as a bench press or squat rack or, in the case of the Olympic lifts, an Olympic lifting bar, bumpers, and a platform that creates a safe area on which to perform the exercises. In contrast, most dumbbell exercises require only an open space for training, a rubber mat or piece of plywood to protect the floor, and an adjustable exercise bench.

Another practical benefit of dumbbell training is that little training space is required, both for storing the dumbbells and for exercising with them. Compare this to machine training, where multiple machines are required to train the entire body, and barbell training, where training occurs with an 8-foot-long (2.4 m) barbell and a recommended 2-foot (61 cm) cushion of space on either end of the barbell. Because of their small size, dumbbells require very little space during training. While you do want a safe buffer around an athlete training with dumbbells, it is possible to train more athletes in a smaller area than could train on either machines or with barbells. Because of the small space requirement during dumbbell training, several athletes can train simultaneously and efficiently with minimal risk of injury. For example, it is possible to have 20 to 25 athletes training with dumbbells in a relatively small area (i.e., 500 square feet) during a training session (broken into groups of two, with one athlete lifting and a partner spotting while waiting to perform a set).

A relatively small number of dumbbells is required to train the entire body. For most people, a weight range from 5 pounds (9.1 kg) to 70 pounds (31.7 kg) in 5-pound (2.3 kg) increments will provide the resistance required to perform most exercises, although some advanced male athletes may need dumbbells 125 pounds (56.7 kg) or heavier. With this limited number of dumbbells it is possible to train all of the major muscle groups of the body performing only dumbbell exercises. For fixed-weight dumbbells (nonadjustable), a weight range from 5 pounds to 70 pounds would require 14 pairs of dumbbells with the weight increasing at 5 pound increments. For adjustable-weight dumbbells, having six 10-pound plates, two 5-pound plates, and two 2 1/2-pound plates would be sufficient to cover a weight range of 5 to 70 pounds (the exact combination would depend on the weight of both the handle and the clamps).

Another benefit of dumbbells is that they are safer than barbells when performing certain exercises, such as one-leg squats or lateral box cross-overs because dumbbells are easier to drop safely than a barbell. Say you are performing one-leg squats and you lose your balance—it is easy to safely drop dumbbells held at arm's length in either hand to regain your balance. However, with a barbell across your back, it is more difficult to drop the barbell safely without risking injury to yourself or to someone standing nearby or damaging the equipment.

Dumbbell training also makes it easier for people with injuries to continue to train without aggravating the injury site. An athlete with an arm or shoulder injury would not be able to train the upper body using a barbell. However, it is possible to perform one-arm dumbbell training using the uninjured arm and continue to train. Similarly, a lower-body injury would prevent athletes from performing Olympic lifts with a barbell. However, by using just one dumbbell, stabilizing the body by holding onto something stable with the opposite hand, and lifting the injured leg off the floor, athletes can adapt the Olympic lifts to accommodate one leg.

A final practical benefit of dumbbell training is that, generally, dumbbell exercises are easier to teach than barbell exercises. For example, most strength and conditioning coaches agree that on average it is much easier to teach someone how to correctly catch a dumbbell clean than to teach that same person how to catch a barbell clean. This means you can get through the teaching process and on to productive training more rapidly when training with dumbbells. This is especially important when working with large groups.

PHYSIOLOGICAL ADVANTAGES OF DUMBBELLS

Several physiological advantages of dumbbell training make it effective. Because barbell training is much more common than dumbbell training, the belief exists that barbell training is superior. A study comparing muscle activation while performing barbell bench press and dumbbell bench press found that the pectoralis major appeared to reach approximately the same peak activation level during the lifting phase of these two chest exercises. While greater muscle recruitment was not demonstrated in the dumbbell movement as compared with the barbell movement as has been suggested by some, this may have occurred because of the low number of repetitions and the low weight used in the study (subjects performed three repetitions with a resistance representing a six-repetition maximum) did not result in fatiguing contractions in the recruited muscles (Welsch et al. 2005).

Perhaps one of the most significant benefits to dumbbell training is that you have to control two independent implements rather than controlling a barbell with both arms simultaneously. This makes dumbbell training a more complex motor activity when performing many exercises.

Because you are working with two independent implements, you have the opportunity to perform either alternating movements (e.g., alternating bench press, with one arm pressing a dumbbell up while the opposite arm is lowering a dumbbell) or single-arm movements (e.g., one-arm bench press, doing all the repetitions with the same arm). For many athletes, alternating-arm exercises and single-arm exercises provide a more sport-specific way to train because many activities in sports involve single-arm movements (e.g., throwing a punch, spiking a volleyball, swinging a racket) rather than both arms moving simultaneously through the same movement pattern (Behm et al. 2011). Further, athletes rarely apply force against a balanced resistance during competition. Both alternating and single-arm movements provide a unique training stimulus compared with typical barbell training (Lauder and Lake 2008).

As a result of controlling two independent implements and the added balance requirement, the stabilizing muscles, which protect the joints, are more active when performing dumbbell training than barbell or machine training. Think of the muscles surrounding the shoulder joint when performing a dumbbell bench press. The stabilizing muscles have to keep the dumbbells in the correct position while preventing them from entering any of the possible incorrect planes of movement. Therefore, dumbbell training can reduce the potential for injury by enhancing joint stability.

Further, keeping the dumbbells stable during an exercise requires increased core muscle activity. It is well accepted that a strong trunk is required for optimal athletic performance. Therefore, training with dumbbells provides an advantage over training with equipment that requires less stabilization and therefore less core muscle recruitment (Koshida et al. 2008).

Working with two separate implements rather than a barbell increases the potential range of motion on certain exercises. For example, when performing a bench press with a bar, the range of motion stops once the bar touches the chest. When using dumbbells, the hands can move lower than the chest because there is no bar to limit the movement.

Dumbbells also add variation to the training program. This is important for both physiological and psychological reasons. Physiologically, variation can help keep the level of stress to the body high during training. The body learns to adapt to the stress of exercise, becoming better able tolerate physical stressors. Because the body adapts quickly to stress, an athlete's goal is to keep the level of stress at the optimal level, and one way to accomplish this is to provide variation in the training program. Frequent variation in exercises requires the body to adapt to a variety of regularly changing stresses applied to the body.

For many athletes, monotony is one of the aspects of training they find most difficult to overcome. This is compounded by performing the same exercises with the same equipment day after day and week after week. Adding dumbbells to the training program increases training variation significantly and reduces psychological staleness.

CONCLUSION

Incorporating dumbbells into your training program offers several advantages. Some of these advantages are practical (e.g., cost, efficient use of space), while some of the advantages have more to do with physiological and psychological benefits. However, when all of the benefits are considered, there is little doubt that both athletes and people training for general fitness should include dumbbells in their training programs.

CHAPTER 2

Designing a Program

Designing effective resistance training programs is critical for achieving optimal results. You can use great technique and train with great intensity, but unless you follow a program that has been well thought out, you will never achieve the best results. Writing a well-designed resistance training program may seem like a daunting task at first. This is, at least in part, because there are so many options and variables to consider. However, with some thought and planning, you can simplify the process into a manageable task.

DETERMINING YOUR PHILOSOPHY OF TRAINING

Although there are several considerations, the most important step in designing training programs is to first establish a philosophy of training. You must determine which training approach best matches your beliefs, based on available research, and then design your training programs based on these beliefs. For example, my philosophy centers around resistance training to develop explosiveness and athleticism, so my resistance training approach is based on free-weight training, emphasizing the Olympic-style exercises such as the snatch, clean, and jerk, which use nearly all of the major muscle groups in the body. In addition to traditional barbell training, I also integrate extensive dumbbell training into my athletes' workouts, taking advantage of the benefits dumbbells provide, which was discussed in chapter 1. While I continue to adjust and tweak the workouts every year, even after 20 years of working as a strength and conditioning coach, I have used this approach for most of my career. I have found an approach I believe in and have stayed with it while continuously trying to improve the product I provide to my athletes. I have said this for a long time, but if I ever get to the point where I feel the workout is as good as it can be, that no further improvements can be made, that is when I need to retire.

BASING TRAINING PROGRAMS ON BOTH SCIENCE AND EXPERIENCE

Develop a philosophy you believe in, one that is based both on science and practical experience. This may sound odd, but the science of strength and conditioning is not at a point where anyone can say that their approach is correct and everyone else is incorrect. As evidence of this, if you were to ask five strength and conditioning coaches to write a program for a specific sport, you would get five different programs. They might be similar in many ways, but they would not be identical.

This is the interesting part of designing training programs because it is part science and part art, art in the sense that you can use your creativity to design what you believe is the best approach to improving athletic performance. Although the art aspect provides room for creativity, the vast majority of a training program should be based on science. A tremendous amount of scientific literature is available to provide you with solid guidelines on developing effective training programs, and it is your responsibility to become familiar with this information so that you can be confident that the training programs you design are scientifically sound.

Basing your workouts on science requires regularly reading peer-reviewed journals and textbooks that are primarily aimed toward the field of exercise science. This eliminates most sources of information that you would find online (unless it is a website for a professional journal) or magazines that you would purchase in a grocery store.

PERIODIZATION

Periodization is the practice of dividing training into specific cycles, with each cycle targeting a specific physiological adaptation. The topic of periodization by itself could make up a textbook, so what follows is a quick review. There are various approaches to periodization. Classical periodization, which is used for a power sport, typically uses the following sequence of training cycles:

1. **Introduction**—Low-volume, low-intensity training prepares athletes for the more demanding training to follow.
2. **Hypertrophy**—High-volume, moderately intense training increases muscle size and muscle endurance. Increasing muscle size is important because of the positive relationship between muscle size and strength.
3. **Strength**—Moderate-volume, high-intensity training begins to bring strength to a peak because of the relationship between strength and power.
4. **Power**—Low-volume, high-intensity training shifts the increases in strength to increases in power.
5. **In-season**—Low-volume, high-intensity training maintains gains in muscle size, strength, and power during the competitive season.

Periodization for a power and endurance sport (e.g., soccer) takes a slightly different approach from the classical style. For example, after the power cycle, a power and endurance cycle of high-volume, moderately intense training that focuses on explosiveness to increase power and endurance simultaneously should be added. The in-season cycle maintains muscle size, strength, power, and endurance through low-volume, high-intensity training.

1. **Introduction**—Low-volume, low-intensity training prepared athletes for the more demanding training to follow.
2. **Hypertrophy**—High-volume, moderately intense training increases muscle size and muscle endurance. Increasing muscle size is important because of the positive relationship between muscle size and strength.
3. **Strength**—Moderate-volume, high-intensity training begins bringing strength to a peak because of the relationship between strength and power.
4. **Power**—Low-volume, high-intensity training shifts the increases in strength to increases in power.
5. **Endurance and power**—High-volume, moderately intense training with an emphasis on explosiveness to increases power and endurance simultaneously.
6. **In-season**—Low-volume, high-intensity training maintains the increases in muscle size, strength, power, and endurance during the competitive season.

The specific cycles, sequences of cycles, and the length of each cycle vary based on training goals, athlete's age and training background, physiological needs of the athlete, and so on. To achieve specific physiological adaptations in each cycle requires carefully manipulating the following training variables.

Rest Times

The length of the rest taken between sets and exercises significantly affects the adaptations that occur through training. Rest times are largely based on the training load. The heavier the load, the longer the rest needs to be. Rest times should be based on the goals of training as demonstrated below:

Training goal	Rest time
Strength	2-5 min
Power	2-6 min
Hypertrophy	30-90 sec
Muscular endurance	30 sec or less

Intensity

Training intensity, or the amount of weight lifted, is based on the training goal. For example, when training for hypertrophy, a higher number of repetitions (e.g., 8-12) are typically performed. Therefore, training intensity must be reduced to allow the athlete to complete the repetitions. In contrast, when training for strength, fewer repetitions (e.g., 1-6) are performed and intensity increases. Training intensity is most frequently expressed as a percentage of a one-repetition maximum (1RM), the most weight a person can lift at one time. Training intensity guidelines are provided in table 2.1.

Table 2.1 Training Intensity Guidelines

Training goal		Load (% 1RM)	Goal repetitions
Strength		>85%	≤6
Power	Single-movement event	80-90%	1-2
	Multiple-effort event	75-85%	3-5
Hypertrophy		65-85%	6-12
Muscle endurance		<65%	>12

Exercise Selection

A variety of resistance training exercises are available, so it is important to choose the exercises best suited to helping you achieve your performance goals. Exercise selection is based on age and maturity, training background, injury status, training goals, and equipment availability.

Age

To develop strength and exercise technique, younger or less mature athletes should start with simple exercises that are less technically demanding. While initially you might consider using exercise machines, be aware that children may be too small to correctly fit the equipment. You might also consider using a barbell, but often the barbell is too heavy for young athletes, so they are unable use correct technique to perform some exercises. Therefore, dumbbells make a great training tool. There is no concern about proper fit and, the lightest dumbbells often weigh 5 pounds (2.3 kg) or less.

Dumbbell training is also appropriate at the opposite end of the age spectrum. Although elderly people usually fit an exercise machine, they may find even the lightest weights too heavy to safely and correctly perform the exercise. The same is true of barbells. Dumbbells, again, are a safe and effective alternative.

Training Background

Athletes with little or no background in resistance training should begin by performing simple exercises. Gradually, as athletes become more experienced, they can choose exercises that are more technically demanding (e.g., cleans vs. power cleans), or exercises that allow more weight to be lifted. On the other hand, someone with an extensive background can train with more demanding, more technically challenging exercises (e.g., overhead lunges vs. lunges). More technically challenging exercises work across several joints, and therefore work nearly the entire body. Not only do these exercises recruit more muscle groups, but they also can more easily result in injury if performed incorrectly.

Injury Status

Exercise choice is affected by injury status. An injured athlete will choose exercises that avoid aggravating the injury site during training. Depending on the severity of the injury, this may dramatically affect exercise selection.

Training Goals

Exercise selection is largely based on training goals. For example, someone training for general fitness may choose machine training, and a body-builder would perform lots of single-joint isolation exercises (e.g., biceps curls) because of the priority on maximal muscle hypertrophy. Because the movements found in sports take place across several joints (e.g., running, jumping, throwing) and power is a key to success, a competitive athlete would choose standing multiple-joint exercises that emphasize speed of movement, typically performed with free weights.

Equipment Availability

Equipment availability also affects exercise selection. The equipment available in your place of training determines the exercises you can perform.

Exercise Order

Although there are exceptions, the following guidelines determine exercise order:

- Perform explosive multijoint exercises (e.g., clean) before exercises performed at a slower speed (e.g., squats). Explosive multijoint exercises require the most energy and emphasis on technique, so they need to be performed before fatigue sets in.

- Perform multiple-joint exercises that target large muscle groups (e.g., deadlift) before single-joint exercises that target smaller muscle groups (e.g., leg extension). Exercises that target large muscle groups require greater energy and focus on technique than do exercises that train small muscle groups.
- Perform single-joint exercises that target small muscle groups (e.g., triceps extension) last. These exercises require the least amount of energy and are less technically difficult.

Number of Sets

Someone with little or no training background can make significant increases in strength by performing a single-set program. However, as training continues, this same person will gain even more strength by performing multiple sets. Multiple sets are beneficial when maximal increases in strength and power is the goal. However, the value of performing more than three sets is minimal; increases in strength when performing four to six sets is not much greater than when performing three sets. On the other hand, when small differences in performance can make a significant difference in competitiveness, performing more than three sets can still be of value. Most highly trained strength and power athletes (e.g., weightlifters, powerlifters) routinely perform four to six sets or more during the majority of their training.

Number of Repetitions

The number of repetitions directly affects both the intensity of training and the energy system called on during training. As the assigned number of repetitions decreases, the training load can increase. As a result, when training for power (1-5 repetitions) or strength (<6 repetitions) a low number of repetitions are performed to allow high-intensity training. In contrast, as the number of repetitions increases, the emphasis can shift to hypertrophy (6-12 repetitions) or muscular endurance (>12 repetitions).

Frequency of Training

The frequency of training depends on the needs of the athlete and the goals of training and varies depending on the specific training cycle. For example, during the off-season, a football offensive lineman might perform resistance training four or five times a week while a soccer player, because of the lower strength demands of the sport, might perform resistance training just twice a week. During the season, when the goal of training shifts from building strength and power to maintaining those qualities, the lineman's training frequency may decrease to once or twice a week.

SAMPLE PROGRAM

Let's use collegiate soccer as an example as I take you through the step-by-step process of designing a training program. Soccer is a fall sport at the collegiate level, with practice beginning in early August and the season running into November or December as teams advance into the playoffs.

This information about the length of the season provides important details. First, it indicates the start date for off-season training. It is generally recommended to provide athletes with at least two weeks off from training to recover physically and psychologically from the demands of competition. At the collegiate level, the athletes will have difficultly training consistently during finals and winter break. So, rather than resuming off-season training in November, only to face interruptions during finals and winter break, it makes more sense to resume training early in January. The start of practice in August signals the end of the off-season phase. With the start and end dates of off-season training established, the number of weeks devoted to off-season training can be determined. Using a typical academic calendar and accounting for a week off at spring break, approximately 28 weeks of off-season training will be available.

Energy Demands

The next variable to determine is the energy demands of the sport. Soccer, except for the goalies, is an endurance and power sport. This is in contrast, for example, to throwing a discus, which is predominantly a power sport, and running a marathon, which is an endurance sport. Studies have shown that, depending on the level of play, the distance covered during a typical soccer game can range from 1.1 to 6 miles based on the age, competition level, and position of the athlete (1.8-10K) (Wang 1995). Because the game involves minimum stoppages of play for brief intervals, the endurance component is quite high.

But rather than requiring continuous slow running, the game is made up of a series of sprints, followed by slower running or walking. This is where the power component is important. At critical times, the soccer player needs to be able to perform with speed and power to make the plays that will determine the outcome of the match.

Determining Sequence of Training Cycles

In collegiate soccer each match is of equal importance (in contrast to a sport like track or swimming, where athletes peak for a specific meet). Therefore, it is important to try to bring the soccer players to a peak in endurance and power just before the start of the season so that they are ready to play at a high level from game one and then maintain that peak for the duration of the season. I know that I have 28 weeks of off-season training and that off-season training will conclude with a cycle designed to maximally increase endurance and power because of the need to peak physically for the start of the competitive phase.

After completion of the in-season phase, the athletes have several weeks off from organized resistance training. They begin off-season training in a detrained state. The off-season training should begin with a brief intro-duction cycle made up of low-volume, low-intensity training to minimize muscular soreness. So, the off-season training begins with an introduction cycle and concludes with an endurance and power cycle.

It is advantageous to first increase strength levels when the goal of training is to develop maximum power because of the positive relation-ship between strength and power. Further, to increase strength it is most effective to first increase muscle mass because of the positive relationship between muscle size and strength. The introduction cycle is followed by a hypertrophy cycle to increase muscle mass before attempting to increase strength levels. After increasing muscle mass, you need to increase strength (because of the relationship between strength and power), so you will place a strength cycle at this point. After increasing strength, you focus on increasing power to improve performance. After increasing power, you conclude off-season training with a cycle to increase endur-ance and power. The sequence of cycles and the length of each cycle could look like this:

Introduction—4 weeks

Hypertrophy—6 weeks

Strength—6 weeks

Power—6 weeks

Endurance and power—6 weeks

Improving the Plan

This progression will accomplish the goal of increasing endurance and power and makes use of the 28 weeks of off-season training. But some aspects of this plan could be improved. First, the goal of training is to provide a constant stress to the body. The body attempts to minimize this stress through adaptation, and the body is proficient at adapting rapidly. Thus, shorter training cycles will provide more frequent adjustments in the training protocol, providing a more consistent level of stress to the body. The advantage of this is that the body is forced to continue to adapt to the stress of training.

Another potential problem with this sequence of cycles is that each cycle (excluding the introduction cycle) is six weeks long, which would indicate that each physiological adaptation (e.g., hypertrophy, strength) is of equal importance in achieving optimal performance in soccer. But I don't believe this is an accurate reflection of the demands of the sport. For example, is increasing muscle mass in a soccer player as important as increasing endurance and power? Increasing muscle mass is of value so that strength can be more effectively increased. But for soccer players, I want to place more emphasis on increasing endurance and power than on increasing muscle mass.

Because of these two factors I want to emphasize the cycles that will have a greater impact on performance. Thus, I prefer the following sequence of cycles:

Introduction—1 week

Hypertrophy—3 weeks

Strength 1—3 weeks

Strength 2—3 weeks

Power—4 weeks

Hypertrophy (repeated)—3 weeks

Strength 2 (repeated)—3 weeks

Endurance and power 1—4 weeks

Endurance and power 2—4 weeks

Sample Workouts

The more refined cycle sequence provides more frequent adjustments in the training protocol, keeping the stress on the body high and also places the greatest emphasis on increasing power and endurance. Now that I have the length and sequence of each cycle organized, I can go back and manipulate the training variables in each cycle to help achieve the desired goal. The first cycle of the training year is a brief introductory cycle. Remember that this training program is based on my own philosophy of training and that a variety of effective techniques can be used to train athletes.

Introduction Cycle

Length   1 week

Goals   Reintroduce athletes to the demands of resistance training and emphasize exercise technique.

Intensity   Complete the full number of repetitions in good form on each set before increasing resistance.

Pace   Perform total-body lifts as explosively as possible. For all other exercises lift in 3 seconds and lower in 3 seconds.

Rest   Take 2:00 between sets and exercises.

Sets and Reps

Week	Introductory cycle
1	TB = 3 × 6 CL = 3 × 8

Tuesday	Thursday
TOTAL BODY	
Clean (mid-shin/floor) TB	Push press TB
LOWER BODY	
Squat CL	Lunge CL
SLDL CL	Lateral squat CL
TRUNK	
Crunch	Twist crunch
Back extension	Twist back extension
UPPER BODY	
Bench press CL	Incline press CL
Row CL	Upright row CL

Note: The following abbreviations are used in the workout tables. TB = total body, one of the Olympic-style lifts or related training exercise; CL = core lift, a multijoint exercise such as a squat; TL = timed lift, the athlete completes the required reps in a specified time; AL = auxiliary lift, a single-joint exercise such as a biceps curl; WT = weighted, the exercise uses external resistance to increase training intensity; MB = medicine ball, the exercise is performed with a medicine ball (medicine balls are often used in training programs when the goal of training is to develop power, because medicine balls are designed to be thrown explosively); RDL = Romanian dead lift; SLDL = straight-leg deadlift; alt = the exercise is performed alternating legs or alternating arms. Starting a DB exercise from the "floor" means beginning the movement from the same position as when using full size weight plates attached to a barbell that is resting on the floor. It is basically a mid-shin position.

The introduction cycle reacquaints the athletes with the demands of resistance training. The full number of repetitions in each set determines the intensity. The athletes select a resistance that allows them to complete the full number of repetitions in each set using good form, forcing them to use a moderate resistance. In some of the later cycles, the first set determines the intensity. The athletes select a resistance they can lift for the full number of repetitions on the first set and perhaps the second set, but if the resistance is selected correctly, they should not be able to complete the full number of repetitions in subsequent sets. The pace, or speed of movement, used during the introduction cycle is relatively slow; whereas, the rest periods between sets and exercises are fairly long.

Exercise selection should be based on training movements, not muscle groups. When resistance training, the increases in strength and power are specific to the movements used to perform the exercise. The more similar the exercise activity is to the movements that make up the sport, the more carryover there will be from the weight room to the playing field. With soccer players I use the resistance training program to increase athleticism instead of simply increasing strength. Therefore, I limit nearly every exercise to dumbbell training. Dumbbells require more balance and body control than machine or barbell exercises do. The goal of training is to improve athletic performance, not improve the ability to demonstrate strength in the weight room.

Exercise selection, similar to program design, should progress from general to specific. As the off-season progresses, exercises should become more and more specific to the movements that occur during competition. For example, it makes sense to perform a basic Olympic-style exercise such as the push press during the introductory cycle to develop strength and teach correct movement patterns. But as the off-season progresses, exercises should also progress. So in the endurance and power cycle that occurs just before the start of practice, the athletes perform split alternating-foot, alternating-arm jerks, which develop power, coordination, and balance.

In terms of exercise order, the Olympic-style exercises are always performed first for two reasons. First, these exercises are performed quickly. Training speed is compromised if athletes go into these exercises fatigued. Second, these exercises involve complex movement patterns, and the ability to perform complex movement patterns diminishes as fatigue sets in. After performing the Olympic-style exercises, athletes perform exercises for the largest muscle groups. In these workouts, the lower body is trained on both training days, so the lower-body exercises are performed after the total-body exercises. These lower-body exercises require lots of energy, so it makes sense to perform these exercises while energy levels are still high.

After athletes have performed the lower-body exercises, they train the trunk. Typically, trunk exercises come at the end of the workout. But a strong trunk is critical for optimal athletic performance, and it has been my experience that if athletes perform trunk training at the end of the workout, many of them will not perform the exercises with the desired intensity. Athletes can perform these trunk exercises with the desired intensity if they do them in the middle of the workout rather than at the end.

Athletes perform the exercises for smaller muscle groups (e.g., chest, shoulders) at the end of the workout, when energy levels are lower. These exercises can be performed safely in a fatigued state. After athletes complete the introduction cycle, they begin the hypertrophy cycle.

Hypertrophy Cycle

Length   3 weeks

Goal   Increase muscular hypertrophy because of the positive relationship between muscle size and strength.

Intensity   Complete the full number of repetitions in good form on each set before increasing resistance.

Pace   Perform total-body lifts as explosively as possible. For all other exercises lift in 3 seconds and lower in 4 seconds.

Rest   Take 1:30 between total-body exercises and 1:00 between all other sets and exercises.

Sets and Reps

Week	Hypertrophy cycle
1	TB = 3 × 6 CL = 3 × 12
2	TB = 3 × 4 CL = 3 × 10
3	TB = 3 × 6 CL = 3 × 12

Tuesday	Thursday
TOTAL BODY	
Clean/squat TB	Front squat/push press TB
Plyometric box jump 3 × 6	Plyometric lateral box jump 3 × 6
LOWER BODY	
Lunge CL	Front squat CL
Superset*: side lunge and leg curl CL	Superset*: side lunge and leg curl CL
Stabilization 1 × 60 sec (each leg)**	
TRUNK	
WT V-up 3 × 25	Twisting crunch 3 × 25
CHEST AND UPPER BODY	
Superset: bench press CL and incline press CL	Superset: bench press CL and incline press CL
SUPERSET	
Superset: row CL and upright row CL	Superset: row CL and upright CL

* A superset occurs when two strength training exercises are performed back-to-back, without rest.

**In the stabilization exercise, the athlete stands on one leg and closes his or her eyes. A partner pushes or pulls the athlete with enough force that the athlete is forced to hop to regain balance. The partner will circle the athlete and push or pull the athlete for the entire 60 seconds of the exercise. The athlete should regain body control and stability before being pushed or pulled each time.

To emphasize increases in muscle size, several variables have been manipulated. First, we reduced the speed of movement to extend the duration of the training stimulus. Next, we increased the number of repetitions and reduced the rest periods because performing resistance training with high repetitions and short rest intervals increases testosterone and human growth hormone levels, both of which are important in muscle growth. Note that the number of repetitions performed varies each week. For example, during weeks 1 and 3 the athletes perform core lifts at 3 × 12, but during week 2 they perform 3 × 10. Because athletes select their resistance based on the required number of repetitions, adjusting the repetitions forces the athletes to vary the training resistance, and thus vary the intensity of their training. In addition, supersets were introduced into the training protocol because of their positive effect on hypertrophy.

Strength Cycle 1

Length 3 weeks

Goal Increase muscular strength because of the positive relationship between strength and power.

Intensity Complete the full number of repetitions in good form on the first set only before increasing resistance.

Pace Perform total-body lifts as explosively as possible. In all other exercises lift in 2 seconds and lower in 2 seconds.

Rest Take 2:00 between all sets and exercises.

Sets and Reps

Week	Strength cycle 1
1	TB = 3 × 4 CL = 3 × 6
2	TB = 3 × 2 CL = 3 × 4
3	TB = 3 × 4 CL = 3 × 6

Tuesday	Thursday
TOTAL BODY	
Clean (shin) TB	Split alt foot jerk TB
Complex: pyramid box jump 3 × 3	Complex: pyramid lateral box jump 3 × 3
LOWER BODY	
One-leg squat CL	Lunge CL
SLDL CL	Side lunge CL
TRUNK	
MB decline crunch throw 3 × 12	MB decline twist 3 × 12
Stabilization 1 × 60 sec (each leg)	
CHEST AND UPPER BODY	
Bench press CL	Seated row CL

In a complex exercise, the individual first performs a resistance training movement (i.e., clean), followed immediately without rest by a plyometric movement. The individual then rests the prescribed time prior to initiating the next set.

After completing the hypertrophy cycle, I have scheduled two consecutive strength cycles. Plyometric exercises are also included in this training cycle. Plyometric exercises are movements that emphasize muscle lengthening (eccentric contraction) followed immediately by muscle shortening (concentric contraction) and are used to help develop muscular power. For example, a common plyometric exercise involves stepping off a box and dropping into a semi-squat position (resulting in an eccentric contraction of the quadriceps) and then immediately jumping off the floor as high and as quickly as possible (resulting in a concentric contraction of the quadriceps). Plyometric exercises have been shown to be effective at helping to develop muscular power.

Strength Cycle 2

Length 3 weeks

Goal Increase muscular strength because of the positive relationship between strength and power.

Intensity Complete the full number of repetitions in good form on the first set only before increasing resistance.

Pace Perform total-body lifts as explosively as possible. In all other exercises lift in 2 seconds and lower in 2 seconds.

Rest Take 2:00 between all sets and exercises.

Sets and Reps

	Strength cycle 2
1	TB = 3 × 3 CL = 3 × 4 AL = 3 × 5
2	TB = 3 × 2 CL = 3 × 2 AL = 3 × 5
3	TB = 3 × 3 CL = 3 × 4 AL = 3 × 5

Tuesday	Thursday
TOTAL BODY	
Alternating-foot split snatch TB	Hang clean TB
Complex: pyramid box jump 3 × 3	Complex: pyramid lateral box jump 3 × 3
LOWER BODY	
One-leg squat CL	Lunge CL
RDL CL	Leg curl AL
Stabilization 1 × 60 sec (each leg)	
TRUNK	
MB stand twist throw 3 × 12	Press crunch 3 × 12
CHEST AND UPPER BACK	
Bench press CL	Row CL

These two strength cycles maximize increases in strength before initiating the first power cycle. To switch the emphasis from hypertrophy to strength, we increased the speed of movement and rest periods and reduced the number of repetitions. These manipulations allow a greater training intensity. Plyometric drills, introduced during these strength cycles, assist in increasing speed, quickness, and agility. During the first two strength cycles, plyometric drills are performed before resistance training movements, so the emphasis can be on high-intensity, high-quality work.

Beginning with strength cycle 1, plyometric training is complexed, meaning the athlete moves immediately from a resistance training movement to a plyometric movement without rest. During a soccer match, athletes compete in a fatigued state and yet must have the ability to move explosively during the critical moments of the game. Complexed training mimics the demand of moving explosively while fatigued.

Power Cycle

<u>**Length**</u>   4 weeks

<u>**Goal**</u>   Increase muscular power because of the positive relationship between power and performance.

<u>**Intensity**</u>   On all lifts complete the full number of repetitions in good form on the first set only before increasing resistance.

<u>**Pace**</u>   Perform total-body lifts as explosively as possible. Perform timed lifts at a pace that allows completion of the full number of required repetitions in the specified time.

<u>**Rest**</u>   Take 2:00 between all sets and exercises.

Sets and Reps

Week	Power cycle
1	TB = 3 × 4 @ 70% TB = 3 × 4 TL = 3 × 8 @ 10 sec CL = 3 × 8
2	TB = 3 × 6 @ 60% TB = 3 × 6 TL = 3 × 10 @ 13 sec CL = 3 × 10
3	TB = 3 × 4 @ 70% TB = 3 × 4 TL = 3 × 8 @ 10 sec CL = 3 × 8
4	TB = 3 × 6 @ 60% TB = 3 × 6 TL = 3 × 10 @ 13 sec CL = 3 × 10

Tuesday	Thursday
TOTAL BODY	
Hang clean TB	Alt split jerk TB
Complex: pyramid box jump 3 × 3	Complex: pyramid lateral box jump 3 × 3
LOWER BODY	
Squat TL	Side lunge TL
TRUNK	
SLDL CL	MB crunch throw 3 × 12
Stabilization 1 × 60 sec	WT twist back extension 3 × 10
CHEST AND UPPER BACK	
Incline press TL	Pull-down CL

The primary manipulations to the workout during the power cycle are the introduction of percentage and timed exercises. Power is a combination of speed and force development or the performance of work expressed per unit of time. Because power is a combination of speed and force, we emphasize speed development during the first workout of the week and force development during the second workout of the week.

Percentages are assigned to the total-body exercises to allow faster movement. It has been determined that highest power outputs occur at 30 percent of one-repetition maximum. The percentages assigned gradually decrease during the power cycles to allow a gradual increase in movement speed. In timed exercises the athlete must complete the exercise in a certain amount of time. Athletes lift as heavy as they can while still completing the required number of repetitions in good form within the time allotted. This shifts the emphasis away from how much they can lift to how quickly they can lift it.

After this power cycle, athletes repeat the hypertrophy and strength 2 cycles. This allows them further gains in muscle size and strength before starting the two consecutive endurance and power cycles that complete off-season training.

Endurance and Power Cycle 1

Length   4 weeks

Goal   Increase muscular power because of the positive relationship between power and performance.

Intensity   On all lifts complete the full number of repetitions in good form on each set before increasing resistance.

Pace   Perform total-body lifts as explosively as possible. Perform timed lifts at a pace that allows completion of the full number of required repetitions in the specified time.

Rest   Take 1:30 between all sets and exercises.

Sets and Reps

Week	Endurance and power cycle 1
1	TB = 3 × 4 @ 70% TB = 3 × 4 TL = 3 × 8 @ 10 sec CL = 3 × 8
2	TB = 3 × 6 @ 60% TB = 3 × 6 TL = 3 × 10 @ 13 sec CL = 3 × 10
3	TB = 3 × 4 @ 70% TB = 3 × 4 TL = 3 × 8 @ 10 sec CL = 3 × 8
4	TB = 3 × 6 @ 60% TB = 3 × 6 TL = 3 × 10 @ 13 sec CL = 3 × 10

Tuesday	Thursday
TOTAL BODY	
Split alt-feet alt snatch TB	Alt split alt jerk TB
Complex: pyramid box jump 3 × 3	Complex: pyramid lateral box jump 3 × 3
LOWER BODY	
Lunge TL (total reps)	Jump lunge TL
Lateral squat TL	Side lunge TL
TRUNK	
MB speed rotation 3 × 18	MB stand twist throw 3 × 18
Stabilization 1 × 60 sec	SLDL 3 × 12
CHEST AND UPPER BACK	
Incline press TL	Pull-down TL

Endurance and Power Cycle 2

Length 4 weeks

Goal Increase muscular power because of the positive relationship between power and performance.

Intensity On all lifts complete the full number of repetitions in good form on each set before increasing resistance.

Pace Perform total-body lifts as explosively as possible. Perform timed lifts at a pace that allows completion of the full number of required repetitions in the specified time.

Rest Take 1:30 between all sets and exercises.

Sets and Reps

Week	Endurance and power cycle 2
1	TB = 3 × 5 @ 60% TB = 3 × 5 TL = 3 × 12 @ 12 sec TL = 3 × 12
2	TB = 3 × 7 @ 50% TB = 3 × 7 TL = 3 × 15 @ 18 sec CL = 3 × 15
3	TB = 3 × 5 @ 60% TB = 3 × 5 TL = 3 × 12 @ 12 sec CL = 3 × 12
4	TB = 3 × 7 @ 50% TB = 3 × 7 TL = 3 × 15 @ 18 sec CL = 3 × 15

Tuesday	Thursday
TOTAL BODY	
Squat alt clean TB	Split alt-foot alt jerk TB
Complex: pyramid box jump 3 × 4	Complex: pyramid lateral box jump 3 × 4
LOWER BODY	
One-leg squat TL	Side lunge TL
Leg curl AL	Stabilization 1 × 60 sec
TRUNK	
Standing speed rotation 3 × 20	MB decline crunch throw 3 × 20
WT back extension 3 × 15	SLDL 3 × 12
UPPER BODY	
Row TL	Bench press TL

To bring the athletes to a peak before the competition phase, I scheduled two consecutive endurance and power cycles. The energy demands of soccer combine the need for endurance and power. To shift the training emphasis to building endurance, we increased the number of repetitions and reduced the rest period between sets and exercises. To maintain the emphasis on power development, we continued the timed lifts to stress the rate of force development.

The exercises mimic movements that make up a soccer game. At the end of the second endurance and power cycle, the athletes are at their peak of physical preparedness. With the start of practice, the focus in the weight room shifts to maintaining this physical peak. Because the athletes are spending a great deal of time and energy in practice, we reduced the number of exercises within the workout and the number of repetitions per set.

Competition

Length   6 weeks

Goal   Maintain increases in muscular endurance and power because of their positive relationship with performance.

Intensity   Complete the full number of repetitions in good form on each set before increasing resistance.

Pace   Perform total-body lifts as explosively as possible. Perform timed lifts at a pace that allows completion of the full number of required repetitions in the specified time.

Rest   Take 1:30 between total-body exercises and 1:00 between all other sets and exercises.

Sets and Reps

Week	Competition 1
1	TB = 3 × 4 TB = 3 × 4 TL = 3 × 10 @ 10 sec
2	TB = 3 × 6 TB = 3 × 6 TL = 3 × 7 @ 9 sec
3	TB = 3 × 4 TB = 3 × 4 TL = 3 × 10 @ 10 sec
4	TB = 3 × 6 TB = 3 × 6 TL = 3 × 7 @ 9 sec
5	TB = 3 × 4 TB = 3 × 4 TL = 3 × 10 @ 10 sec
6	TB = 3 × 6 TB = 3 × 6 TL = 3 × 7 @ 9 sec

Monday	Wednesday
TOTAL BODY	
Alt hang clean TB	Split alt-foot alt jerk TB
LOWER BODY	
Squat TL	Side lunge TL
Leg curl TL	
TRUNK	
MB one-leg twist throw 3 × 10	Decline crunch press 3 × 10
WT twist back extension 3 × 8	
Stabilization 1 × 60 sec	
CHEST AND UPPER BACK	
Bench press TL	Pull-down TL

Plyometric training is eliminated; the athletes are running, jumping, cutting, stopping, and starting as a part of practice and competition. Attempting to practice daily, compete twice per week, perform resistance training twice per week, and participate in plyometric training twice per week has the potential to lead to overtraining. The emphasis must be directed to on-field activities during this time, and other forms of training become secondary.

CONCLUSION

Designing effective resistance training programs is a critical task for the strength and conditioning coach. For athletes to reach their peak performance capabilities, they need a scientifically based strength and conditioning program. It is the responsibility of the strength and conditioning coach to provide his or her athletes with the best possible program to help them achieve their performance goals. Although designing a high-quality training program is a time-consuming process, your athletes deserve the time and effort it takes to design a superior program for them. Designing an effective resistance training program is critical if you are to reach your peak performance capabilities. You need a scientifically based strength and conditioning program that will help you achieve your performance goals. Although designing a high-quality training program is time consuming, it is worth the effort.

CHAPTER 3

Incorporating Dumbbells Into an Existing Program

Taking an existing program and incorporating dumbbells into it is normally an easy process because nearly every barbell- or machine-based exercise can also be performed with dumbbells. What is more difficult is deciding how much of the existing program you want to convert to dumbbell-based training and which dumbbell-specific variations you want to introduce into the training program now that the option exists.

Determining how much of an existing program you want to convert to dumbbell training should be based on several factors. First, what are the demands of the sport? If your sport and position within that sport require a lot of strength, for example an offensive lineman in football, you might want to keep the emphasis on barbell training while adding variety through dumbbell training. This is because, quite simply, you can use more weight in a barbell exercise than you can with a dumbbell exercise. For example, an offensive lineman may be able to bench press 300 pounds (136 kg). To lift an equal amount of weight with dumbbells would require the athlete to use 150-pound (68 kg) dumbbells, which would be considered highly extraordinary. In some athletic training facilities, 150-pound dumbbells can be found, but their use, especially when performing a DB bench, would be far out of the norm.

This is not to suggest that an offensive lineman should avoid dumbbell training altogether. Dumbbells provide unique advantages over other forms of training. However, the athlete would emphasize barbell training while still taking advantage of the benefits that dumbbells provide. In my own situation as the head strength and conditioning coach at Colorado State University at Pueblo, I design the strength training program for the football team so that the players in the big skill positions (offensive and defensive line, tight ends, and linebackers) perform resistance training three times per week. Two of those weekly workouts are barbell orientated while one workout per week emphasizes dumbbell training. Success in these positions requires a high level of strength and power, so we emphasize barbell training to maximize the increases in muscle size and strength while supplementing this with a dumbbell-training day.

In contrast, the skill position players (quarterbacks, running backs, wide receivers, defensive backs, and kickers) also train three times per week, but the emphasis is reversed. These groups train with dumbbells twice per week and train with barbells once per week. While strength and power are important for success in these positions, movement skills and athleticism are also important. Therefore, I emphasize dumbbell training with these athletes (while still including barbell training) to develop the coordination, balance, and motor skills their positions require. Both the big skill and skill positions perform barbell cleans, squats, and bench press (or associated training exercises) twice a week, once with a barbell and once with dumbbells.

My soccer players, on the other hand, train exclusively with dumbbells. The strength demands for soccer are less than they are for football. However, the technical demands in soccer are extremely high. It is definitely a sport that requires a high level of balance, coordination, agility, and motor skills. Emphasizing dumbbell training exclusively with this group makes sense.

Program design and exercise selection vary based not only on the sport and the position played but also on the frequency that dumbbell training is performed. For example, with football players in big skill positions, who train with dumbbells just once per week, each dumbbell training day provides a full-body workout. Players perform a dumbbell Olympic lift to start the workout, they next train the lower body with dumbbell exercises, perform a trunk exercise, and then they train the upper body with dumbbells. Because they only train with dumbbells once per week, I want them to receive the benefits of training with dumbbells in both the lower and upper body. In contrast, the skill position players emphasize the lower body on one of their dumbbell-training days, emphasize the upper body on the other dumbbell-training day (while starting both workouts performing a dumbbell Olympic lift), and train both the lower and upper body on their barbell day. Using this method, both groups train the lower body and upper body twice per week, once with a barbell and once with a dumbbell. Soccer players, because the strength demands for their sport are lower, perform strength training just twice per week and train all of the major muscle groups in the body during both workouts.

I also periodize exercise selection, progressing from basic exercises early in the off-season to more demanding and complex exercises as the off-season progresses. This emphasizes motor skills as the competitive season draws nearer. So, for example, athletes begin off-season training by performing a dumbbell push press, advance to a power jerk during the next cycle, progress to a split alternating-foot jerk, and then finish the off-season by performing an alternating-arm, alternating-foot split jerk.

Although the process of taking an existing workout and converting it to a dumbbell workout is fairly straightforward, a lot of thought goes into developing the workout plan based on the demands of the sport and the specific training cycle you are developing.

SAMPLE WORKOUTS WITH BARBELLS

The first workout presented is for softball players that predominantly use barbells. The primary emphasis of this training plan is to increase muscle size (i.e., hypertrophy) and the secondary emphasis is to increase strength. The training variables (e.g., rest times, pace, intensity) are also labeled depending on the training goal. So the rest times when the goal is hypertrophy are shorter than when the goal is to build strength, because shorter rest times are recommended for increasing muscle size and longer rest times are recommended for increasing strength.

You will also notice that the pitchers perform more repetitions than the field players on a majority of the exercises. This difference is because the endurance demands are greater for the pitchers than for the field players. To build endurance, pitchers perform more repetitions.

Hypertrophy and Strength Cycle: Barbells

Monday

Length 5 weeks

Goal Begin increasing muscle size because of the positive relationship between muscle size and strength.

Intensity Hypertrophy and strength: Select a resistance that allows completion of all the repetitions in each set before increasing resistance.

Pace Perform total-body lifts as explosively as possible. Hypertrophy: Lower in 3 seconds. Strength: Lower in 2 seconds.

Rest Hypertrophy: Take 1:30 between total-body sets and exercises and 1:00 between all other sets and exercises. Strength: Take 2:00 between sets and exercises.

Sets and Reps

Week	Strength: field players*	Strength: pitchers*
1	TB = 4 × 4 CL = 3 × 8	TB = 4 × 4 CL = 3 × 9
2	TB = 4 × 4 CL = 3 × 8	TB = 4 × 4 CL = 3 × 9
3	TB = 4 × 4 CL = 3 × 8	TB = 4 × 4 CL = 3 × 9
4	TB = 4 × 4 CL = 3 × 8	TB = 4 × 4 CL = 3 × 9
5	TB = 4 × 4 CL = 3 × 8	TB = 4 × 4 CL = 3 × 9

*Strength: Perform all reps in each set.

	Week 1	Week 2	Week 3	Week 4	Week 5
TOTAL BODY					
Clean TB	4 × 4 + 4 × 4	4 × 2 + 4 × 2	4 × 4 + 4 × 4	4 × 2 + 4 × 2	4 × 2
Weight lifted					
LOWER BODY					
Squat CL	3 × 8-7-6 + 3 × 9-8-7	3 × 5-4-3 + 3 × 7-6-5	3 × 8-7-6 + 3 × 9-8-7	3 × 5-4-3 + 3 × 7-6-5	3 × 5-4-3
Weight lifted					
SLDL CL Squat CL	3 × 8-7-6 + 3 × 9-8-7	3 × 5-4-3 + 3 × 7-6-5	3 × 8-7-6 + 3 × 9-8-7	3 × 5-4-3 + 3 × 7-6-	3 × 5-4-3
Weight lifted					
UPPER BODY					
Bench press CL	3 × 8-7-6 + 3 × 9-8-7	3 × 5-4-3 + 3 × 7-6-5	3 × 8-7-6 + 3 × 9-8-7	3 × 5-4-3 + 3 × 7-6-5	3 × 5-4-3
Weight lifted					
TRUNK					
Kneeling plate twist	3 × 15	3 × 15	3 × 15	3 × 15	3 × 12
Weight lifted					
ROTATOR CUFF					
Empty can	2 × 12	2 × 12	2 × 12	2 × 12	2 × 12
Weight lifted					

Note: The following abbreviations are used in the workout lists. TB = total body, one of the Olympic-style lifts or related training exercise; CL = core lift, a multijoint exercise such as a squat; alt = the exercise is performed alternating legs or alternating arms.

Wednesday

Length 5 weeks

Goal Begin increasing muscle size because of the positive relationship between muscle size and strength.

Intensity Hypertrophy and strength: Select a resistance that allows completion of all the repetitions in each set before increasing resistance.

Pace Perform total-body lifts explosively. Hypertrophy: Lift as explosively as possible and lower in 3 seconds. Strength: Lift as explosively as possible and lower in 2 seconds.

Rest Hypertrophy: Take 1:30 between total-body sets and exercises and 1:00 between all other sets and exercises. Strength: Take 2:00 between sets and exercises.

Sets and Reps

Week	Strength: field players*	Strength: pitchers*
1	TB = 4 × 4 CL = 3 × 8	TB = 4 × 4 CL = 3 × 9
2	TB = 4 × 4 CL = 3 × 8	TB = 4 × 4 CL = 3 × 9
3	TB = 4 × 4 CL = 3 × 8	TB = 4 × 4 CL = 3 × 9
4	TB = 4 × 4 CL = 3 × 8	TB = 4 × 4 CL = 3 × 9
5	TB = 4 × 4 CL = 3 × 8	TB = 4 × 4 CL = 3 × 9

*Strength: Perform all reps in the first set.

	Week 1	Week 2	Week 3	Week 4	Week 5
TOTAL BODY					
Clean TB	4 × 4 + 4 × 4	4 × 2 + 4 × 2	4 × 4 + 4 × 4	4 × 2 + 4 × 2	4 × 2
Weight lifted					
LOWER BODY					
Squat CL	3 × 8-7-6 + 3 × 9-8-7	3 × 5-4-3 + 3 × 7-6-5	3 × 8-7-6 + 3 × 9-8-7	3 × 5-4-3 + 3 × 7-6-5	3 × 5-4-3
Weight lifted					
SLDL CL	3 × 8-7-6 + 3 × 9-8-7	3 × 5-4-3 + 3 × 7-6-5	3 × 8-7-6 + 3 × 9-8-7	3 × 5-4-3 + 3 × 7-6-5	3 × 5-4-3
Weight lifted					
UPPER BODY					
Bench press CL	3 × 8-7-6 + 3 × 9-8-7	3 × 5-4-3 + 3 × 7-6-5	3 × 8-7-6 + 3 × 9-8-7	3 × 5-4-3 + 3 × 7-6-5	3 × 5-4-3
Weight lifted					
TRUNK					
Kneeling plate twist	3 × 15	3 × 15	3 × 15	3 × 15	3 × 12
Weight lifted					
ROTATOR CUFF					
Empty can	2 × 12	2 × 12	2 × 12	2 × 12	2 × 12
Weight lifted					

(continued)

Hypertrophy and Strength Cycle: Barbells *(continued)*

Friday

Length 5 weeks

Goal Begin increasing muscle size because of the positive relationship between muscle size and strength.

Intensity Hypertrophy and strength: Select a resistance that allows the completion of all the repetitions on each set before increasing resistance.

Pace Perform total-body lifts explosively. Hypertrophy: Lift as explosively as possible and lower in 3 seconds. Strength: Lift as explosively as possible and lower in 2 seconds.

Rest Hypertrophy: Take 1:30 between total-body sets and exercises and 1:00 between all other sets and exercises. Strength: Take 2:00 between sets and exercises.

Sets and Reps

Week	Hypertrophy: field players*	Hypertrophy: pitchers*	Strength: field players	Strength: pitchers
1	TB = 4 × 5 CL = 3 × 10	TB = 4 × 5 CL = 3 × 12	TB = 4 × 4 CL = 3 × 8	TB = 4 × 4 CL = 3 × 9
2	TB = 4 × 3 CL = 3 × 8	TB = 4 × 3 CL = 3 × 10	TB = 4 × 4 CL = 3 × 8	TB = 4 × 4 CL = 3 × 9
3	TB = 4 × 5 CL = 3 × 10	TB = 4 × 5 CL = 3 × 12	TB = 4 × 4 CL = 3 × 8	TB = 4 × 4 CL = 3 × 9
4	TB = 4 × 3 CL = 3 × 8	TB = 4 × 3 CL = 3 × 10	TB = 4 × 4 CL = 3 × 8	TB = 4 × 4 CL = 3 × 9
5	TB = 4 × 2 CL = 3 × 6	TB = 4 × 2 CL = 3 × 6	TB = 4 × 4 CL = 3 × 8	TB = 4 × 4 CL = 3 × 9

*Hypertrophy: Perform all reps in each set.

	Week 1	Week 2	Week 3	Week 4	Week 5
TOTAL BODY					
Power jerk TB	4 × 5	4 × 3	4 × 5	4 × 3	4 × 2
Weight lifted					
CHEST					
Incline press CL	3 × 10 + 3 × 12	3 × 8 + 3 × 10	3 × 10 + 3 × 12	3 × 8 + 3 × 10	3 × 6
Weight lifted					
Pull-down CL	3 × 10 + 3 × 12	3 × 8 + 3 × 10	3 × 10 + 3 × 12	3 × 8 + 3 × 10	3 × 6
Weight lifted					
Stabilization	1 × 45 sec	1 × 45 sec	1 × 45 sec	1 × 60 sec	1 × 45 sec
Each leg					
TRUNK					
Decline two-plate twist	3 × 15 + 3 × 20	3 × 15 + 3 × 20	3 × 15 + 3 × 20	3 × 15 + 3 × 20	3 × 12
Weight lifted					
ROTATOR CUFF AND SCAPULA					
Functional rotation	2 × 12	2 × 12	2 × 12	2 × 12	2 × 12
Weight lifted					
Prone overhead thumbs-up lateral raise	2 × 12	2 × 12	2 × 12	2 × 12	2 × 12
Weight lifted					

SAMPLE WORKOUTS WITH DUMBBELLS

The next three workouts are nearly identical to the previous three. The goals and the variables that make up the training plan are the same. However, the exercises in the following workouts have been adjusted so that the training is done mostly with dumbbells rather than barbells.

Hypertrophy and Strength Cycle: Dumbbells

Monday

Length 5 weeks

Goal Begin increasing muscle size because of the positive relationship between muscle size and strength.

Intensity Select a resistance that allows completion of all of the repetitions in each set before increasing resistance.

Pace Perform total-body lifts explosively. In all other exercises lift as explosively as possible and lower in 3 seconds.

Rest Take 1:30 between total-body sets and exercises and 1:00 between all other sets and exercises.

Sets and Reps

Week	Strength: field players*	Strength: pitchers*
1	TB = 4 × 5 CL = 3 × 10	TB = 4 × 5 CL = 3 × 12
2	TB = 4 × 3 CL = 3 × 8	TB = 4 × 3 CL = 3 × 10
3	TB = 4 × 5 CL = 3 × 10	TB = 4 × 5 CL = 3 × 12
4	TB = 4 × 3 CL = 3 × 8	TB = 4 × 3 CL = 3 × 10
5	TB = 4 × 2 CL = 3 × 6	TB = 4 × 2 CL = 3 × 6

*Strength: Perform full reps in each set.

	Week 1	Week 2	Week 3	Week 4	Week 5
TOTAL BODY					
Hang clean TB	4 × 5	4 × 3	4 × 5	4 × 3	4 × 2
Weight lifted					
LOWER BODY					
One-leg squat CL	3 × 10 + 3 × 12	3 × 8 + 3 × 10	3 × 10 + 3 × 12	3 × 8 + 3 × 10	3 × 6
Weight lifted					
Lateral squat CL	3 × 10 + 3 × 12	3 × 8 + 3 × 10	3 × 10 + 3 × 12	3 × 8 + 3 × 10	3 × 6
Weight lifted					
TRUNK					
Alt toe touch	3 × 15 + 3 × 20	3 × 15 + 3 × 20	3 × 15 + 3 × 20	3 × 15 + 3 × 20	3 × 12
Weight lifted					
UPPER BACK					
Row CL	3 × 10 + 3 × 12	3 × 8 + 3 × 10	3 × 10 + 3 × 12	3 × 8 + 3 × 10	3 × 6
Weight lifted					
ROTATOR CUFF AND SCAPULA					
Internal rotation	2 × 12	2 × 12	2 × 12	2 × 12	2 × 12
Weight lifted					
Prone thumbs-up lateral raise	2 × 12	2 × 12	2 × 12	2 × 12	2 × 12
Weight lifted					

(continued)

Hypertrophy and Strength Cycle: Dumbbells *(continued)*

Wednesday

<u>Length</u> 5 weeks

<u>Goal</u> Begin increasing muscle size because of the positive relationship between muscle size and strength.

<u>Intensity</u> Select a resistance that allows completion of all repetitions in each set before increasing resistance.

<u>Pace</u> Perform total-body lifts explosively. Hypertrophy: Lift as explosively as possible and lower in 3 seconds. Strength: Lift as explosively as possible and lower in 2 seconds.

<u>Rest</u> Hypertrophy: Take 1:30 between total-body sets and exercises and 1:00 between all other sets and exercises. Strength: Take 2:00 between sets and exercises.

Sets and Reps

Week	Strength: field players*	Strength: pitchers*
1	TB = 4 × 4 CL = 3 × 8	TB = 4 × 4 CL = 3 × 9
2	TB = 4 × 2 CL = 3 × 8	TB = 4 × 2 CL = 3 × 7
3	TB = 4 × 4 CL = 3 × 8	TB = 4 × 4 CL = 3 × 9
4	TB = 4 × 2 CL = 3 × 8	TB = 4 × 2 CL = 3 × 7
5	TB = 4 × 4 CL = 3 × 8	TB = 4 × 4 CL = 3 × 9

*Strength: Perform full reps in first set.

	Week 1	Week 2	Week 3	Week 4	Week 5
TOTAL BODY					
Clean TB	4 × 4 + 4 × 4	4 × 2 + 4 × 2	4 × 4 + 4 × 4	4 × 2 + 4 × 2	4 × 2
Weight lifted					
LOWER BODY					
Squat CL	3 × 8-7-6 + 3 × 9-8-7	3 × 5-4-3 + 3 × 7-6-5	3 × 8-7-6 + 3 × 9-8-7	3 × 5-4-3 + 3 × 7-6-5	3 × 5-4-3
Weight lifted					
SLDL CL	3 × 8-7-6 + 3 × 9-8-7	3 × 5-4-3 + 3 × 7-6-5	3 × 8-7-6 + 3 × 9-8-7	3 × 5-4-3 + 3 × 7-6-5	3 × 5-4-3
Weight lifted					
UPPER BODY					
Bench press CL	3 × 8-7-6 + 3 × 9-8-7	3 × 5-4-3 + 3 × 7-6-5	3 × 8-7-6 + 3 × 9-8-7	3 × 5-4-3 + 3 × 7-6-5	3 × 5-4-3
Weight lifted					
TRUNK					
Kneeling plate twist	3 × 15	3 × 15	3 × 15	3 × 15	3 × 12
Weight lifted					
ROTATOR CUFF					
Empty can	2 × 12	2 × 12	2 × 12	2 × 12	2 × 12
Weight lifted					

Friday

Length   5 weeks

Goal   Begin increasing muscle size because of the positive relationship between muscle size and strength.

Intensity   Hypertrophy and strength: Select a resistance that allows completion of all repetitions in each set before increasing resistance.

Pace   Perform total-body lifts explosively. Hypertrophy: Lift as explosively as possible and lower in 3 seconds. Strength: Lift as explosively as possible and lower in 2 seconds.

Rest   Hypertrophy: Take 1:30 rest between total-body sets and exercises and 1:00 between all other sets and exercises. Strength: Take 2:00 between sets and exercises.

Sets and Reps

Week	Hypertrophy: field players*	Hypertrophy: pitchers*	Strength: Field players	Strength: pitchers
1	TB = 4 × 5 CL = 3 × 10 AL = 3 × 10	TB = 4 × 5 CL = 3 × 12 AL = 3 × 12	TB = 4 × 4 CL = 3 × 8 AL = 3 × 8	TB = 4 × 4 CL = 3 × 9 AL = 3 × 10
2	TB = 4 × 3 CL = 3 × 8 AL = 3 × 10	TB = 4 × 3 CL = 3 × 10 AL = 3 × 12	TB = 4 × 4 CL = 3 × 8 AL = 3 × 8	TB = 4 × 4 CL = 3 × 9 AL = 3 × 10
3	TB = 4 × 5 CL = 3 × 10 AL = 3 × 10	TB = 4 × 5 CL = 3 × 12 AL = 3 × 12	TB = 4 × 4 CL = 3 × 8 AL = 3 × 8	TB = 4 × 4 CL = 3 × 9 AL = 3 × 10
4	TB = 4 × 3 CL = 3 × 8 AL = 3 × 10	TB = 4 × 3 CL = 3 × 10 AL = 3 × 12	TB = 4 × 4 CL = 3 × 8 AL = 3 × 8	TB = 4 × 4 CL = 3 × 9 AL = 3 × 10
5	TB = 4 × 2 CL = 3 × 6 AL = 3 × 10	TB = 4 × 2 CL = 3 × 6 AL = 3 × 12	TB = 4 × 4 CL = 3 × 8 AL = 3 × 8	TB = 4 × 4 CL = 3 × 9 AL = 3 × 10

*Hypertrophy: Perform full reps in each set.

(continued)

Hypertrophy and Strength Cycle: Dumbbells *(continued)*

	Week 1	Week 2	Week 3	Week 4	Week 5
TOTAL BODY					
Power jerk TB	4 × 5	4 × 3	4 × 5	4 × 3	4 × 2
Weight lifted					
CHEST					
Incline press CL	3 × 10 + 3 × 12	3 × 8 + 3 × 10	3 × 10 + 3 × 12	3 × 8 + 3 × 10	3 × 6
Weight lifted					
Bent lateral raise AL	3 × 10 + 3 × 12	3 × 8 + 3 × 10	3 × 10 + 3 × 12	3 × 8 + 3 × 10	3 × 6
Weight lifted					
Stabilization	1 × 45 sec	1 × 45 sec	1 × 45 sec	1 × 60 sec	1 × 45 sec
Each leg					
TRUNK					
Decline two-plate twist	3 × 15 + 3 × 20	3 × 15 + 3 × 20	3 × 15 + 3 × 20	3 × 15 + 3 × 20	3 × 12
Weight lifted					
ROTATOR CUFF AND SCAPULA					
Functional rotation	2 × 12	2 × 12	2 × 12	2 × 12	2 × 12
Weight lifted					
Prone overhead thumbs-up lateral raise	2 × 12	2 × 12	2 × 12	2 × 12	2 × 12
Weight lifted					

CONCLUSION

In reviewing and comparing the workouts with barbells to the ones with dumbbells, you can see how easy it is to shift the workouts from predominately barbell exercises to predominately dumbbell. Because most barbell exercises can also be performed with dumbbells, in most instances you simply have to indicate that the exercise will be done with dumbbells rather than prescribing a different exercise. The emphasis of the training plan, in this case training for hypertrophy as the primary goal and strength as the secondary goal, does not change when emphasizing dumbbell exercises. The only change is in the equipment.

PART II

EXERCISES

Dumbbells can be used to train all of the major muscle groups in the body. Further, dumbbells provide some unique advantages as compared to strictly training with a barbell. As a result it makes sense to include dumbbells in your training program. Chapters 4 through 7 provide descriptions of a variety of dumbbell exercises. The chapters are broken into upper-body exercises, lower-body exercises, core exercises, and total-body exercises (e.g., cleans, jerks, snatches and their associated variations).

In my job as a collegiate strength and conditioning coach, I stress that exercise technique takes priority over intensity. While I expect my athletes to work very hard, and they do, being able to perform the exercise correctly is always more important than how much weight they use. Technique is priority number one; intensity is priority number two. Therefore, it is important for you to carefully read the exercise descriptions and make sure the positions you use when performing the exercises match the positions shown in the pictures. This is the best way to maximize the time and effort you put into your training program.

CHAPTER 4

Upper Body

The muscles of the upper body are responsible for, or contribute to, a variety of movements involved in athletics, such as throwing, pushing, pulling, and swinging. And it is important to remember that many of the movements that occur in the upper body (e.g., throwing, swinging) originate in the lower body, are transferred through the core, and expressed in the upper body. Therefore, it is important to train both the lower body and the core to maximize many upper-body movements.

Many athletes and people involved in strength training make the mistake of emphasizing upper-body training while neglecting the trunk and lower body. This may be because they associate strength and improved appearance with the size of the biceps and pecs. Training the upper body is important, but athletes should also train the major muscle groups in the trunk and lower body. The body functions most efficiently when sufficient strength has been developed in all of the major muscle groups.

In our discussion of dumbbell exercises to train the upper body, we have divided the upper body into five areas: shoulders, chest, upper back, biceps, and triceps.

SHOULDERS

The primary shoulder muscles are the deltoids. Secondary muscles are the supraspinatus, trapezius, pectoralis major and minor, and latissimus dorsi.

Front Raise

Instructions

1. Hold the dumbbells palms down and with arms straight so that the dumbbells are resting against the top of the thighs.
2. Keeping the elbows locked, and without using a rocking motion at the torso, maintain a palms-down position and lift the dumbbells to shoulder height.
3. Pause for a count and then lower the dumbbells under control to the start position.

Common Errors

- Performing the movement too quickly reduces the amount of time the muscles are under tension, potentially decreasing the training effect.
- Using dumbbells that are too heavy can cause poor technique, such as lifting or lowering too quickly, bending the elbows, or reducing the range of motion. Always emphasize technique over the amount of weight lifted. If you are unable to lift using correct technique, select lighter dumbbells.
- Using a rocking motion at the torso to generate momentum to assist in the lifting action decreases the training effect on the target muscles.

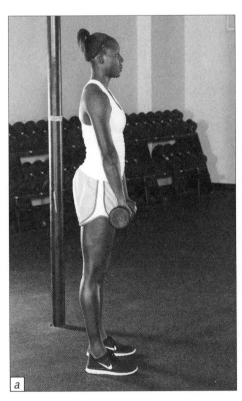
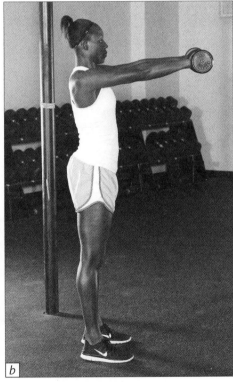

a   b

Lateral Raise

Instructions

1. Hold the dumbbells at your sides with a slight bend at the elbow and the palms facing inward so that the dumbbells are resting against the top of the outside of the thighs.
2. Keeping the elbows slightly bent and without rocking at the torso, maintain a palms-down position and lift the dumbbells laterally to shoulder height.
3. Pause for a count and then lower the dumbbells under control to the start position.

Common Errors

- Performing the movement too quickly reduces the amount of time the muscles are under tension, potentially decreasing the training effect.
- Using dumbbells that are too heavy results in improper technique, such as lifting or lowering too quickly, excessive bending at the elbows, and reduced range of motion.
- Using a rocking motion at the torso to generate momentum and assist in the lifting action decreases the training effect on the target muscles. Do not rock your body to create momentum and make the exercise easier.

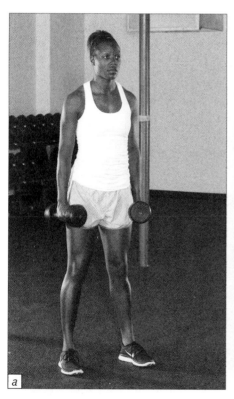

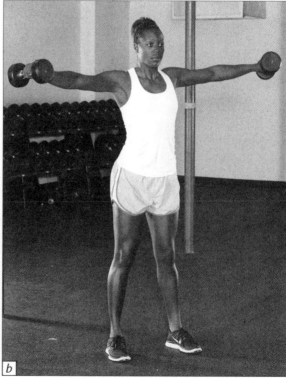

Shoulder Press

Instructions

1. Hold the dumbbells at the shoulders so that the palms face forward and the elbows point toward the ground.
2. Press the dumbbells directly up so that the elbows are completely extended.
3. Do not use the lower body to assist in the lifting action.
4. Do not lean back as you press the dumbbells up. At the top of the movement the shoulders should be directly over the hips.
5. Pause for a count and then lower the dumbbells under control to the start position.

Common Errors

- Performing the movement too quickly reduces the amount of time the muscles are under tension, potentially decreasing the training effect.
- Using dumbbells that are too heavy results in improper technique, such as lifting or lowering too quickly, improper body position, and reduced range of motion.
- Using the lower body to generate momentum assists in the lifting phase of the movement and decreases the training effect on the target muscles.
- Leaning back at the torso while pressing the dumbbells up increases the stress on the lower back. The ankle, knee, hip, and shoulder should all be in a straight line.

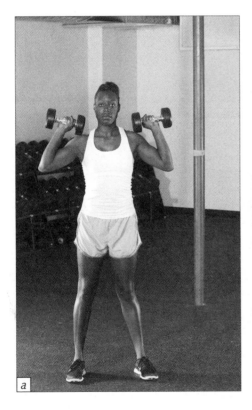
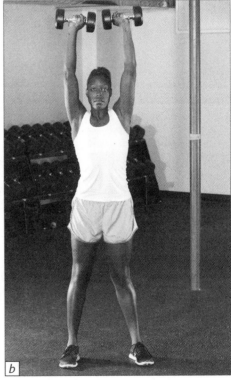

Alternating Shoulder Press

Instructions

1. Hold the dumbbells at the shoulders so that the palms face forward and the elbows point toward the ground.
2. Press the right dumbbell directly upward so that the elbow is completely extended.
3. Do not use the lower body to assist in the lifting action.
4. Do not lean back as you press the dumbbell up. At the top of the movement the shoulders should be directly over the hips.
5. Lower the right dumbbell to the starting point while simultaneously pressing the left dumbbell overhead to a fully extended position.
6. Pause for a count and then lower the left dumbbell to the start position while raising the right dumbbell.

Common Errors

- Performing the movement too quickly reduces the amount of time the muscles are under tension, potentially decreasing the training effect.
- Using dumbbells that are too heavy results in improper technique, such as lifting or lowering too quickly, improper body position, and reduced range of motion.
- Using the lower body to generate momentum to assist in the lifting phase of the movement can decrease the training effect.
- Leaning back at the torso while pressing the dumbbells can create stress on the lower back. The ankle, knee, hip, and shoulder should all be in a straight line.
- Leaning away from the side that is lifting the dumbbell can reduce the training effect. Keep the body in a straight line.

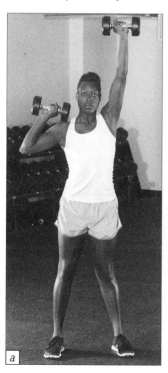 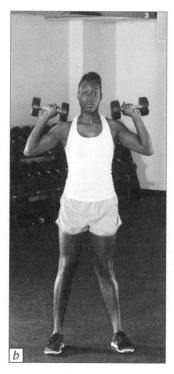 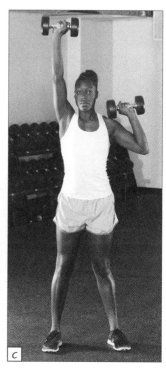

One-Arm Shoulder Press

Instructions

1. Hold one dumbbell at the shoulder so that the palm faces forward and the elbow points toward the ground.
2. Press the dumbbell directly up until the elbow is completely extended.
3. Do not use the lower body to assist in the lifting action.
4. Do not lean back as you press the dumbbell up. At the top of the movement the shoulders should be directly over the hips.
5. Pause for a count and then lower the dumbbell under control to the start position.

Common Errors

- Performing the movement too quickly reduces the amount of time the muscles are under tension, potentially decreasing the training effect.
- Using dumbbells that are too heavy results in improper technique, such as lifting or lowering too quickly, improper body position, and reduced range of motion.
- Using the lower body to generate momentum and assist in the lifting phase of the movement can decrease the training effect.
- Leaning back at the torso while pressing the dumbbells can cause stress on the lower back. The ankle, knee, hip, and shoulder should be in a straight line.
- Leaning away from the side that is lifting the dumbbell can decrease the training effect. Keep the body in a straight line.

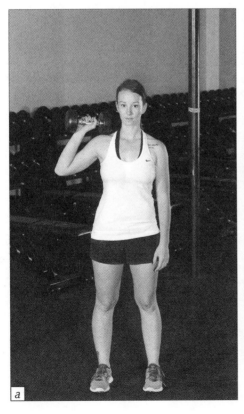
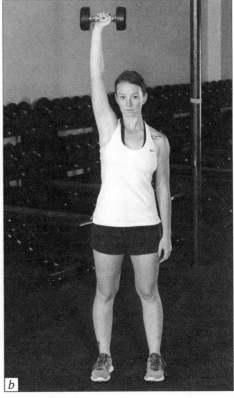

Upright Row

Instructions

1. Hold the dumbbells with straight arms and the palms facing down so that the dumbbells are resting against the top of the thighs.
2. Keeping the elbows above the wrists and the dumbbells orientated laterally, lift the dumbbells to shoulder height.
3. Do not rock the upper body to generate momentum and assist in lifting the dumbbells.
4. Pause for a count and then lower the dumbbells under control to the start position.

Common Errors

- Performing the movement too quickly reduces the amount of time the muscles are under tension, potentially decreasing the training effect.
- Using dumbbells that are too heavy results in improper technique, such as lifting or lowering too quickly, improper body position, and reduced range of motion.
- Allowing the wrist to elevate above the elbow rather than keeping it under the elbow reduces the training effect on the shoulder muscles.
- Using the lower body or a rocking motion of the torso to assist in the lifting of the dumbbells reduces the training effect.

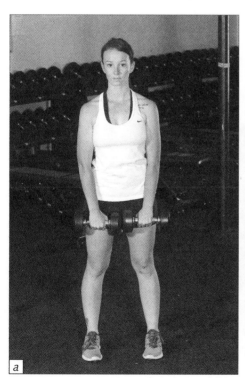
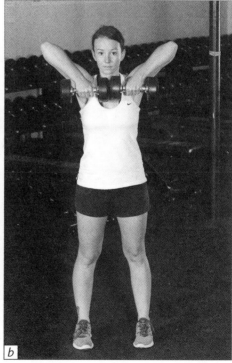

CHEST

The primary muscle of the chest is the pectoralis major. The pectoralis minor is a secondary muscle.

Pullover

Instructions

1. Position yourself on an exercise bench so that the upper back and shoulders are supported by the bench.
2. Bend the knees and place the feet flat on the floor so that the knees, hips, and shoulders are all in a straight line.
3. Turn the dumbbell top to bottom and grasp the dumbbell on the inside face of the weight stack at the top of the dumbbell.
4. Extend the arms so that the dumbbell is positioned at arms' length directly over the face.
5. With just a slight bend at the elbows lower the dumbbells through a full comfortable range of motion until the dumbbell is positioned over the top of the head.
6. Keeping a slight bend at the elbows return the dumbbell to the starting position.

Common Errors

- Performing the movement too quickly reduces the amount of time the muscles are under tension, potentially decreasing the training effect.
- Using dumbbells that are too heavy results in the use of improper technique, such as lifting or lowering too quickly, improper body position, and reduced range of motion.
- Too much bend in the elbows shifts the emphasis away from the muscles of the chest.

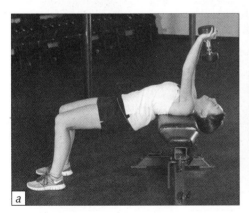
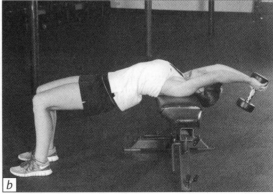

Fly

Instructions

1. Lie faceup on an exercise bench and place the feet flat on the floor.
2. Hold a dumbbell in each hand, straight above the chest, with palms facing each other.
3. With the elbows slightly bent, lower the dumbbells laterally to the level of the rib cage.
4. Maintaining a slight bend in the elbows, lift the dumbbells back to the starting position.

Common Errors

- Performing this movement too quickly reduces the amount of time the muscles are under tension, potentially decreasing the training effect.
- Using dumbbells that are too heavy results in improper technique, such as lifting or lowering too quickly, improper body position, and reduced range of motion.
- Too much bend in the elbows reduces the training effect on the chest.
- Completing less than a full range of motion limits the recruitment of the target muscle group.

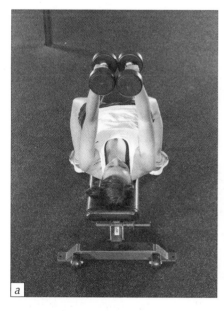
a

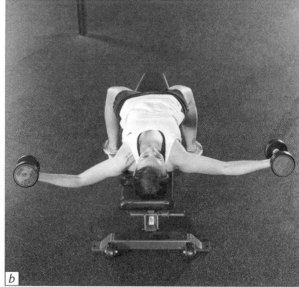
b

Incline Fly

Instructions

1. Lie faceup on an incline exercise bench and place the feet flat on the floor.
2. Hold a dumbbell in each hand, straight above the chest, with palms facing each other.
3. With the elbows slightly bent, lower the dumbbells laterally to the level of the rib cage.
4. Maintaining a slight bend in the elbows, lift the dumbbells back to the starting position.
5. Placing the bench at an incline of 20-30 degrees tends to shift the emphasis to the upper portion of the pectoralis, as compared to performing the exercise on a flat bench.

Common Errors

- Performing this movement too quickly reduces the amount of time the muscles are under tension, potentially decreasing the training effect.
- Using dumbbells that are too heavy results in improper technique, such as lifting or lowering too quickly, improper body position, and reduced range of motion.
- Too much bend in the elbows reduces the training effect on the chest.
- Completing less than a full range of motion limits the recruitment of the target muscle group.

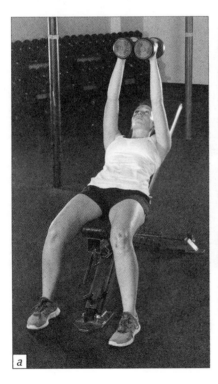
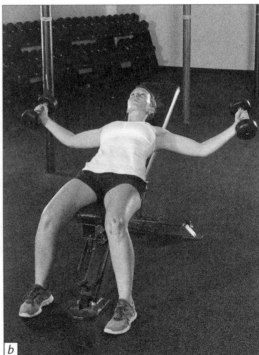

Decline Fly

Instructions

1. Lie face up on a decline exercise bench.
2. Hold a dumbbell in each hand, straight above the chest, with palms facing each other.
3. With the elbows slightly bent, lower the dumbbells laterally to the level of the rib cage.
4. Maintaining a slight bend in the elbows, lift the dumbbells back to the starting position.
5. Placing the bench at a decline of 20-30 degrees tends to shift the emphasis to the mid to lower portion of the pectoralis, as compared to performing the exercise on a flat bench.

Common Errors

- Performing the movement too quickly reduces the amount of time the muscles are under tension, potentially decreasing the training effect.
- Using dumbbells that are too heavy results in improper technique, such as lifting or lowering too quickly, and improper body position.
- Excessive bend at the elbows reduces the training effect on the chest muscles.
- Completing less than a full range of motion limits the recruitment of the target muscle group.

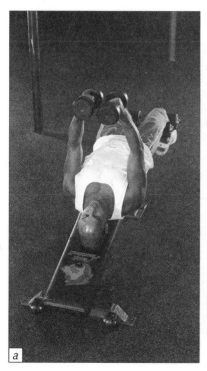
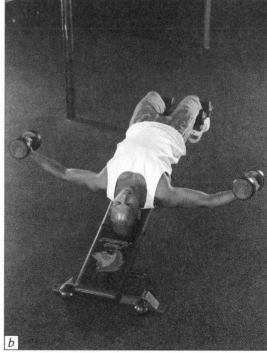

Incline Press

Instructions

1. Lie face up on an incline exercise bench and place the feet flat on the floor.
2. Hold the dumbbells laterally at chest height.
3. Simultaneously press both dumbbells up until both arms are fully extended directly above the shoulders.
4. Lower the dumbbells under control to the start position.

Common Errors

- Performing the movement too quickly reduces the amount of time the muscles are under tension, potentially decreasing the training effect.
- Using dumbbells that are too heavy results in improper technique, such as lifting or lowering too quickly, improper body position, and reduced range of motion.
- Elevating the hips off the bench and excessively arching the low back increase the stress placed on the lower back and decreases the emphasis on the muscles of the chest.
- Completing less than a full range of motion limits the recruitment of the target muscle group.

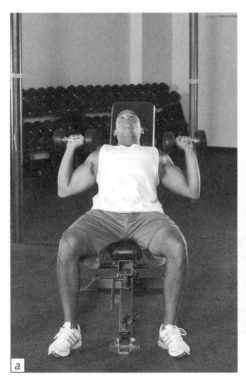
a

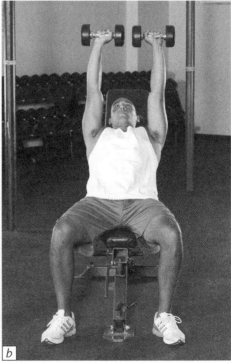
b

Alternating Incline Press

Instructions

1. Lie faceup on an incline exercise bench and place the feet flat on the floor.
2. Hold the dumbbells laterally at chest height.
3. Press the right dumbbell up until the right arm is fully extended directly above the right shoulder. Hold the dumbbell in the left arm motionless.
4. As you lower the right arm repeat the movement with the left arm.
5. On each repetition lower the dumbbell under control to the start position.

Common Errors

- Performing the movement too quickly reduces the amount of time the muscles are under tension, potentially decreasing the training effect.
- Using dumbbells that are too heavy results in improper technique, such as lifting or lowering too quickly, improper body position, and reduced range of motion.
- Elevating the hips off the bench excessively arches the lower back.
- Twisting the upper body as a means to gain leverage when lifting the dumbbell increases the opportunity for injury to the lower back. Keep the hips and shoulders flat on the bench during the exercise.

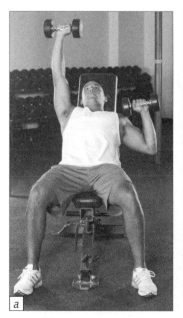
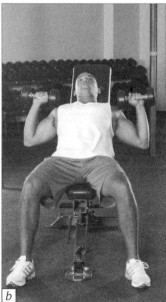
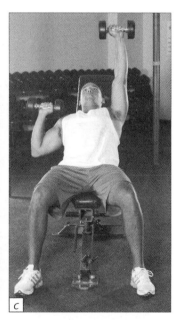

a   b   c

One-Arm Incline Press

Instructions

1. Lie faceup on an incline exercise bench and place the feet flat on the floor.
2. Hold one dumbbell laterally at chest height.
3. Press the dumbbell up until the arm is fully extended directly above the shoulder.
4. Complete the required number of repetitions and then repeat the movement on the other arm.
5. On each repetition lower the dumbbell under control to the start position.

Common Errors

- Performing the movement too quickly reduces the amount of time the muscles are under tension, potentially decreasing the training effect.
- Using dumbbells that are too heavy results in the use of improper technique, such as lifting or lowering too quickly, improper body position, and reduced range of motion.
- Elevating the hips off the bench excessively arches the lower back.
- Twisting the upper body to gain leverage when lifting the dumbbell stresses the lower back.

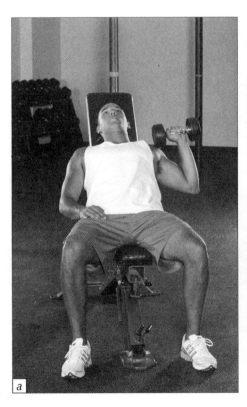 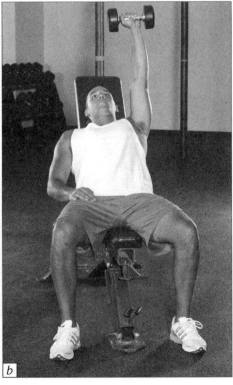

Decline Press

Instructions

1. Lie faceup on a decline exercise bench.
2. Hold the dumbbells laterally at chest height.
3. Simultaneously press both dumbbells up until both arms are fully extended directly above the shoulders.
4. Lower the dumbbells under control to the start position.

Common Errors

- Performing the movement too quickly which reduces the amount of time the muscles are under tension, potentially decreasing the training effect.
- Using dumbbells that are too heavy results in the use of improper technique, such as lifting or lowering too quickly, improper body position, and reduced range of motion.
- Elevating the hips off the bench excessively arches the lower back.
- Limiting the range of motion reduces the training effect.

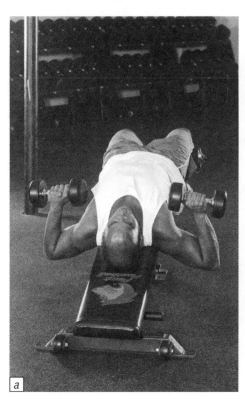

a

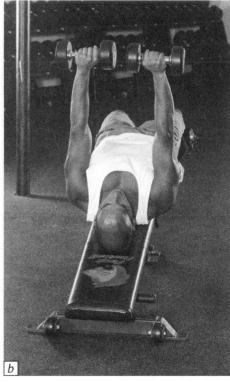

b

Alternating Decline Press

Instructions

1. Lie faceup on a decline exercise bench.
2. Hold the dumbbells laterally at chest height.
3. Press the right dumbbell up until the right arm is fully extended directly above the right shoulder.
4. As you lower the right arm repeat the movement with the left arm.
5. On each repetition lower the dumbbell under control to the start position.

Common Errors

- Performing the movement too quickly reduces the amount of time the muscles are under tension, potentially decreasing the training effect.
- Using dumbbells that are too heavy results in improper technique, such as lifting or lowering too quickly, improper body position, and reduced range of motion.
- Elevating the hips off the bench excessively arches the lower back.
- Twisting the upper body to gain leverage when lifting the dumbbell can stress the lower back.

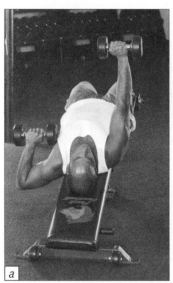 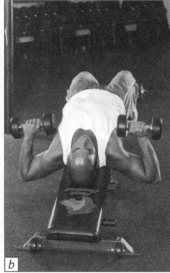 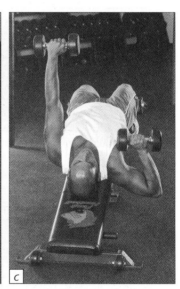

One-Arm Decline Press

Instructions

1. Lie faceup on a decline exercise bench.
2. Hold one dumbbell laterally at chest height.
3. Press the dumbbell up until the arm is fully extended directly above the shoulder.
4. Complete the required number of repetitions and then repeat the movement on the other arm.
5. On each repetition, lower the dumbbell under control to the start position.

Common Errors

- Performing the movement too quickly reduces the amount of time the muscles are under tension, potentially decreasing the training effect.
- Using dumbbells that are too heavy results in improper technique, such as lifting or lowering too quickly, improper body position, and reduced range of motion.
- Elevating the hips off the bench excessively arches the lower back.
- Twisting the upper body to gain leverage when lifting the dumbbell can stress the lower back.

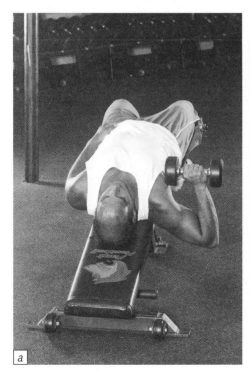
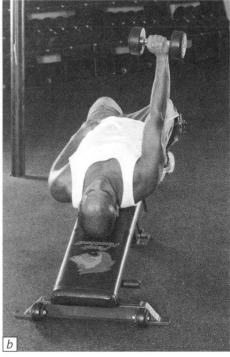

Bench Press

Instructions

1. Lie faceup on an exercise bench and place the feet flat on the floor.
2. Hold the dumbbells laterally at chest height.
3. Simultaneously press both dumbbells up until both arms are fully extended directly above the shoulders.
4. Lower the dumbbells under control to the start position.

Common Errors

- Performing the movement too quickly reduces the amount of time the muscles are under tension, potentially decreasing the training effect.
- Using dumbbells that are too heavy results in improper technique, such as lifting or lowering too quickly or improper body position.
- Limiting the range of motion reduces the training effect.

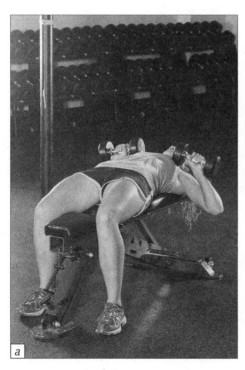
a

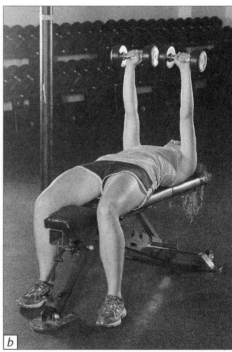
b

Alternating Bench Press

Instructions

1. Lie faceup on an exercise bench and place the feet flat on the floor.
2. Hold the dumbbells laterally at chest height.
3. Press the right dumbbell up until the right arm is fully extended directly above the right shoulder.
4. As you lower the right arm repeat the movement with the left arm.
5. On each repetition lower the dumbbell under control to the start position.

Common Errors

- Performing the movement too quickly reduces the amount of time the muscles are under tension, potentially decreasing the training effect.
- Using dumbbells that are too heavy results in improper technique, such as lifting or lowering too quickly, improper body position, and reduced range of motion.
- Elevating the hips off the bench excessively arches the lower back.
- Twisting the upper body to gain leverage when lifting the dumbbell can stress the lower back.

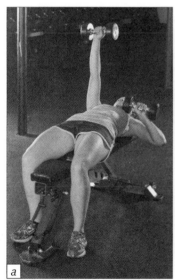
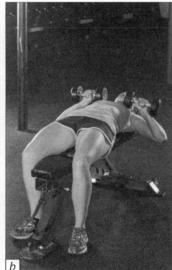
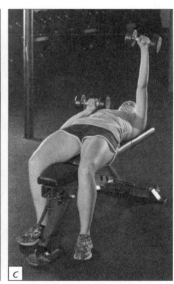

a   b   c

One-Arm Bench Press

Instructions

1. Lie faceup on an exercise bench and place the feet flat on the floor.
2. Hold one dumbbell laterally at chest height.
3. Press the dumbbell up until the arm is fully extended directly above the shoulder.
4. Complete the required number of repetitions and then repeat the movement on the other arm.
5. On each repetition lower the dumbbell under control to the start position.

Common Errors

- Performing the movement too quickly reduces the amount of time the muscles are under tension, potentially decreasing the training effect.
- Using dumbbells that are too heavy results in improper technique, such as lifting or lowering too quickly, improper body position, and reduced range of motion.
- Elevating the hips off the bench excessively arches the lower back.
- Twisting the upper body to gain leverage when lifting the dumbbell can stress the lower back.

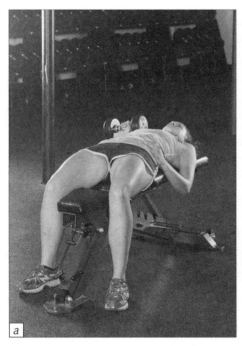

a

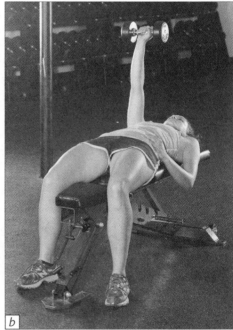

b

UPPER BACK

The primary muscles of the upper back are the latissimus dorsi, rhomboids, and trapezius. The secondary muscles are the rhomboids and teres minor.

Row

Instructions

1. Place the left knee on a flat exercise bench, positioned directly under the left hip.
2. Bend at the hips and lower the trunk until the back is flat and the head is up.
3. With the left palm flat on the bench, fully extend the left arm.
4. Grasp a dumbbell with the right hand, the palm facing the body.
5. Shrug the shoulder toward the ceiling, attempting to lift the dumbbell as high as possible without bending the right elbow.
6. At the top of the shrug bend the right elbow and pull the dumbbell to the outside of the rib cage.
7. Lower the dumbbell under control.
8. Perform the required number of repetitions and then adjust the body position so that the movement can be performed with the left arm.

Common Errors

- Performing the movement too quickly reduces the amount of time the muscles are under tension, potentially decreasing the training effect.
- Using dumbbells that are too heavy results in improper technique, such as lifting or lowering too quickly, improper body position, and reduced range of motion.
- Using a jerking or twisting movement to lift the dumbbell keeps the lifting action from being smooth and controlled.
- Failing to hold the dumbbell in a straight line under the shoulder so that the dumbbell can contact the body toward the outside of the rib cage.

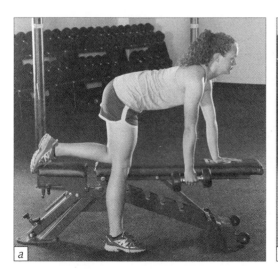
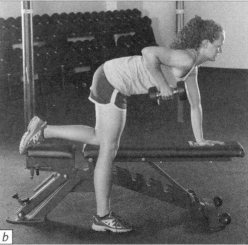

a

b

BICEPS

The primary muscle of the front of the upper arm is the biceps. The secondary muscle is the brachialis.

Curl

Instructions

1. Grasp a pair of dumbbells with a palms-up grip.
2. Extend the arms so that dumbbells are held at thigh height.
3. Without rocking the upper body, curl the dumbbells to a fully flexed position at shoulder height.
4. Lower the dumbbells under control to the start position.

Common Errors

- Performing the movement too quickly reduces the amount of time the muscles are under tension, potentially decreasing the training effect.
- Using dumbbells that are too heavy results in improper technique, such as lifting or lowering too quickly, improper body position, and reduced range of motion.
- Using a rocking motion of the torso to assist in the lifting action decreases the workload on the target muscle group. Although you can lift more weight when you rock, less work is required of the target muscle group, reducing the effectiveness of the exercise.

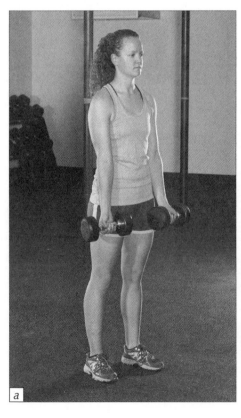
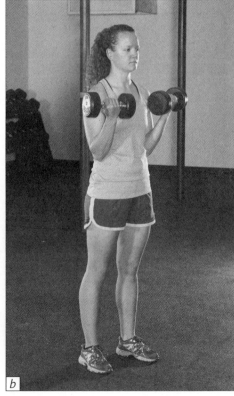

a   b

Hammer Curl

Instructions

1. Hold a pair of dumbbells at thigh height so that the palms face each other and thumbs are up. The feet are shoulder-width apart.
2. Starting with the dumbbells lateral to the thighs, maintain a thumbs-up position and flex at the elbow without rocking the upper body until the dumbbells reach the top position.
3. Lower the dumbbells under control.

Common Errors

- Performing the movement too quickly reduces the amount of time the muscles are under tension, potentially decreasing the training effect.
- Using dumbbells that are too heavy results in improper technique, such as lifting or lowering too quickly, improper body position, and reduced range of motion.
- Using a rocking motion at the torso to assist in lifting reduces the effectiveness of the exercise on the targeted muscle group.

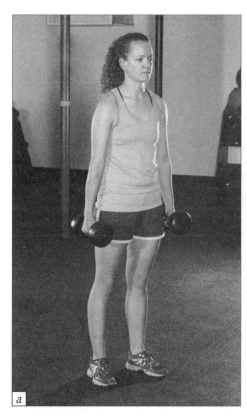
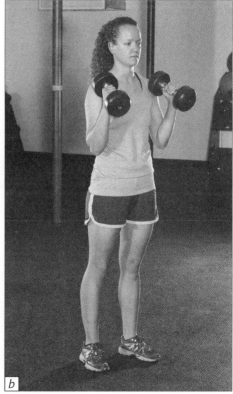

a

b

Reverse Curl

Instructions

1. Grasp a pair of dumbbells with a palms-down grip.
2. Extend the arms so that dumbbells are held at thigh height.
3. Without rocking the upper body and maintaining a palms-down position, curl the dumbbells to a fully flexed position at shoulder height.
4. Lower the dumbbells under control to the start position.

Common Errors

- Performing the movement too quickly reduces the amount of time the muscles are under tension, potentially decreasing the training effect.
- Using dumbbells that are too heavy results in improper technique, such as lifting or lowering too quickly, improper body position, and reduced range of motion.
- Using a rocking motion at the torso to assist in the lifting reduces the effectiveness of the exercise.

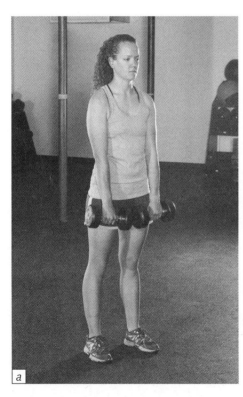
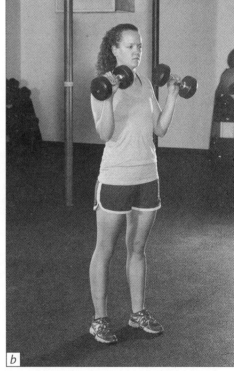

a   b

TRICEPS

The primary muscle of the back of the upper arm is the triceps. The secondary muscle is the anconeus.

Triceps Extension

Instructions

1. Turn a dumbbell on its side.
2. Open the hands and grasp the dumbbell on the inside portion of the top weight stack.
3. Fully extend the arms upward so that the dumbbell is held top to bottom directly over the head.
4. Fully flex the elbows to lower the dumbbell under control behind the head.
5. Extend the elbows to return to the start position.

Common Errors

- Performing the movement too quickly reduces the amount of time the muscles are under tension, potentially decreasing the training effect.
- Using dumbbells that are too heavy results in improper technique, such as lifting or lowering too quickly, using improper body position, and reduced range of motion.
- Rocking the torso to assist in the lifting action reduces the effectiveness of the exercise.
- Letting the elbows drift away from each other instead of keeping them just outside the width of the head decreases the training effect on the target muscles.

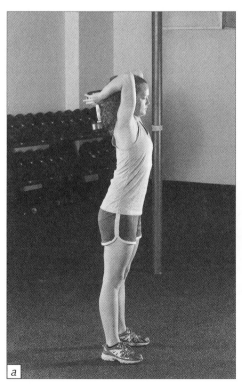
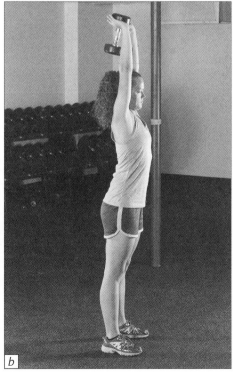

Kickback

Instructions

1. Place the left knee on a flat exercise bench, positioned directly under the left hip.
2. Bend at the hips and lower the trunk until the back is flat. The head is up.
3. Straighten the left arm so that it is fully extended, the left palm flat on the bench supporting the upper body.
4. Grasp a dumbbell with the right hand so that the palm of the right hand faces the body.
5. Flex at the right elbow and shoulder until the right forearm is lifted to the height of the hip.
6. The elbow is bent at a right angle so that the right hand in a straight line below the elbow and is parallel to the right leg.
7. Keeping the upper arm in this position, extend the forearm at the elbow toward the hip until the dumbbell is lifted to the same height as the elbow.
8. Lower the dumbbell under control.

Common Errors

- Performing the movement too quickly reduces the amount of time the muscles are under tension, potentially decreasing the training effect.
- Using dumbbells that are too heavy results in improper technique, such as lifting or lowering too quickly, using improper body position, and not completing the movement through a full range of motion.
- Rocking the torso to assist in the lifting action reduces the effectiveness of the exercise.

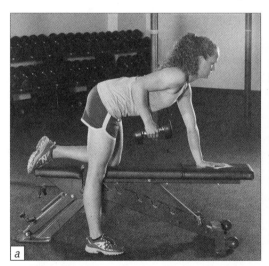
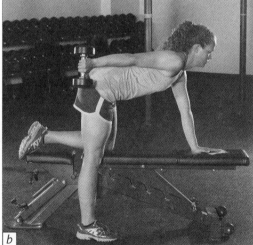

CHAPTER 5

Lower Body

People sometimes have a tendency to emphasize the upper body in strength training programs because they often equate being strong and powerful with having big arms or a big chest. In reality, however, most sports are lower-body dominant. That is, a strong and powerful lower body has much more to do with success in most sports than do big biceps. This chapter discusses a variety of strength and power training exercises for the lower body. The primary muscles in the lower body are the gluteals, hamstrings, adductors, and quadriceps.

Squat

Instructions

1. Grasp a dumbbell in each hand with the arms fully straightened along the sides of the body.
2. Assume a shoulder-width stance.
3. Arch the back, and keep the head up.
4. Maintaining an arched back, initiate the squat movement by sitting back at the hips.
5. Continue to sit back until the thighs are parallel with the floor. The center of the hip joint should be at the same height or below the center of the knee joint.
6. The heels should be on the floor. The knees can drift slightly in front of the toes, in a line directly over the toes or can line up slightly behind the toes depending on what is most comfortable.
7. Leading with the head (as opposed to lifting the hips first) return to the starting position. The back should remain arched and the head should be up.

Common Errors

- Allowing the back to round rather than arching it during the exercise, which places more stress on the low back and can lead to injury.
- Failing to achieve a thigh position that is parallel to the floor at the bottom of the movement.
- Initiating the movement by moving the knees forward rather than by sitting back at the hips, which lifts the heels off the floor.
- Lowering the weight too quickly rather than controlling the movement during the descent.

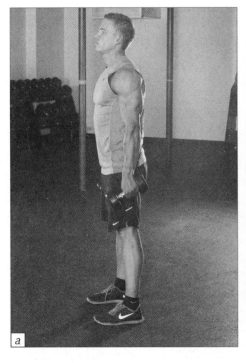
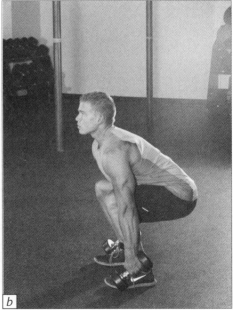

a b

Jump Squat

Instructions

1. Grasp a dumbbell in each hand with the arms fully straightened along the sides of the body.
2. Assume a shoulder-width stance.
3. Arch the back, and keep the head up.
4. Maintaining an arched back, initiate the movement by sitting back at the hips.
5. Continue to sit back until your thigh is at the same depth as in a typical maximal vertical-jump attempt.
6. The heels should be on the floor. The knees can drift slightly in front of the toes in a line directly over the toes or can be slightly behind the toes, depending on what is most comfortable.
7. Leading with the head (as opposed to lifting the hips first), use a jumping action to elevate off the floor. The back should remain arched and the head should be up during this jump phase.

Common Errors

- Allowing the back to round rather than arching it during the exercise, which places more stress on the low back and can lead to injury.
- Failing to achieve the depth of a typical maximal vertical-jump attempt.
- Initiating the movement by moving the knee forward rather than sitting back at the hips, which lifts the heels off the floor.
- Spending too much time on the floor between repetitions rather than executing each jump as quickly as possible.

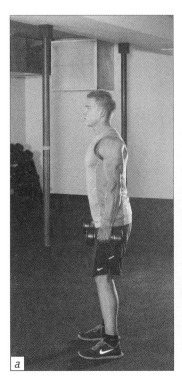
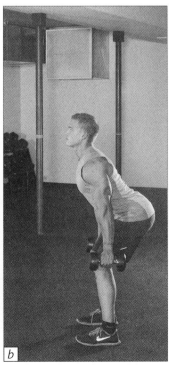
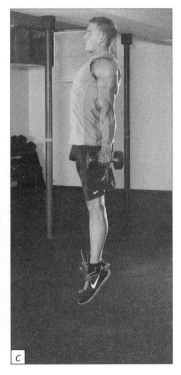

a

b

c

One-Leg Squat

Instructions

1. Grasp a dumbbell in each hand with the arms straight along the sides of the body.
2. Assume a shoulder-width stance.
3. Arch the back, and keep the head up.
4. Reach back with the right leg and place the right foot on a bench or plyometric box that is approximately knee height.
5. The left foot should be far enough in front of the bench that you are in a lunge position.
6. Maintaining an arched back, initiate the movement by sitting back at the hips.
7. Continue to sit back until your left thigh is parallel to the floor. The center of the hip joint should be at the same height as the center of the knee joint.
8. The front heel should stay on the floor. The front knee can drift slightly in front of the toes in a line directly over the toes or line up slightly behind the toes depending on what is most comfortable.
9. Leading with the head (as opposed to lifting the hips first), return to the starting position. The back should remain arched and the head should be up.

Common Errors

- Allowing the back to round rather than maintaining an arch during the exercise.
- Failing to lower until the thigh is parallel to the floor, which is especially common in this exercise.
- Initiating the movement by moving the knee forward rather than sitting back at the hip, which can cause the heels to lift off the floor.
- Lowering the weight too quickly rather than controlling the descent.

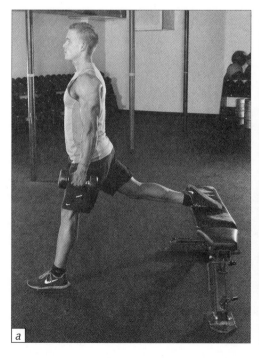 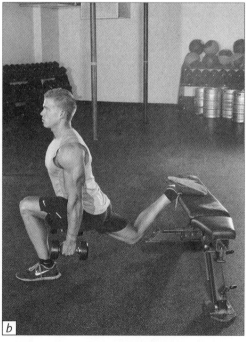

One-Leg Jump Squat

Instructions

1. Grasp a dumbbell in each hand with the arms up at approximately shoulder height.
2. Assume a shoulder-width stance.
3. Arch the back, and keep the head up.
4. Reach back with the right leg and place the right foot on a bench or plyometric box that is approximately knee height.
5. The left foot should be far enough in front of the bench that you are in a lunge position.
6. Maintaining an arched back, initiate the movement by sitting back at the hips.
7. Continue to sit back until your thigh is at the same depth as in a typical maximal vertical-jump attempt.
8. The front heel should be on the floor.
9. The lead knee can drift slightly in front of the toes in a line directly over the toes or lined up slightly behind the toes depending on what is most comfortable.
10. Leading with the head (as opposed to lifting the hips first) use a jumping action to elevate off the floor. The back should remain arched and the head should be up during this jump phase.
11. The back should remain arched, and the head should be up.

Common Errors

- Allowing the back to round rather than maintaining an arch during the exercise.
- Failing to lower the body until the thigh is parallel to the floor.
- Initiating the movement by moving the knee forward rather than by sitting back at the hips, which can raise the heels off the floor.
- Failing to achieving the depth of a typical maximal vertical jump.
- Spending too much time on the floor between repetitions, rather than jumping as quickly as possible.

(continued)

One-Leg Jump Squat *(continued)*

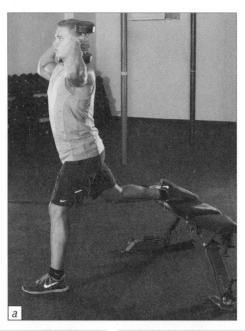

a

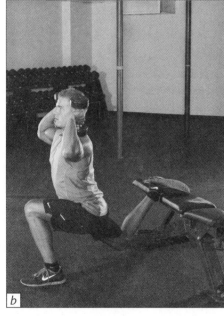

b

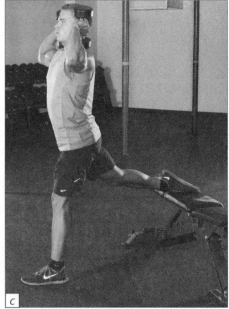

c

Front Squat

Instructions

1. Grasp a dumbbell in each hand with the arms at the sides.
2. Raise the dumbbells to the shoulders, with the back end of the dumbbells resting on the shoulders. Hold the elbows high so that the dumbbells are level. The front end should not be lower than the back end.
3. Assume a shoulder-width stance.
4. Arch the back, and keep the head up.
5. Maintaining an arched back, initiate the movement by sitting back at the hips.
6. Continue to sit back until the thighs are parallel to the floor. The center of the hip joint should be at the same height as the center of the knee joint.
7. The heels should remain on the floor. The knees can drift slightly in front of the toes in a line directly over the toes or line up slightly behind the toes depending on what is most comfortable.
8. Leading with the head (as opposed to lifting the hips first) return to the starting position. The back should remain arched, and the head should be up.

Common Errors

- Allowing the back to round rather than arching it during the exercise. (Keep the elbows high to eliminate this problem.)
- Failing to lower the body until the thigh is parallel to the floor at the bottom of the movement.
- Initiating the movement by moving the knee forward rather than by sitting back at the hips, which can lift the heels off the floor.
- Lowering the weight too quickly rather than controlling the descent.

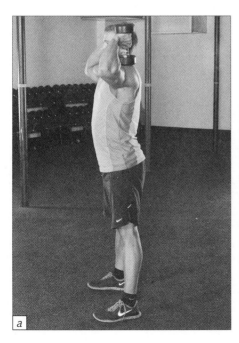
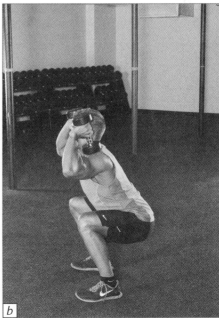

One-Leg Front Squat

Instructions

1. Grasp a dumbbell in each hand with the arms at the sides.
2. Raise the dumbbells to the shoulders, with the back of the dumbbells resting on the shoulders. Hold the elbows high so that the dumbbells are level. Don't let the front of the dumbbells sit lower than the back.
3. Assume a shoulder-width stance.
4. Arch the back, and keep the head up.
5. Reach back with the left leg and place the left foot on a bench or plyometric box that is approximately knee height.
6. The right foot should be far enough in front of the bench that you are in a lunge position.
7. Maintaining an arched back, initiate the movement by sitting back at the hips.
8. Continue to sit back until the thigh is parallel to the floor. The center of the hip joint should be at the same height as the center of the knee joint.
9. The heels should be on the floor. The knees can drift slightly in front of the toes in a line directly over the toes or line up slightly behind the toes depending on what is most comfortable.
10. Leading with the head (as opposed to lifting the hips first) return to the starting position. The back should remain arched, and the head should be up.

Common Errors

- Allowing the back to round rather than arching it during the exercise.
- Failing to lower until the thigh is parallel to the floor.
- Initiating the movement by moving the knee forward rather than by sitting back at the hips, which can lift the heels off the floor.
- Lowering the weight too quickly rather than controlling the descent.

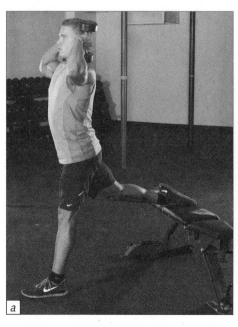 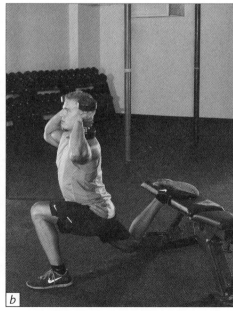

Lateral Squat

Instructions

1. Grasp a dumbbell in each hand, arms straight at the sides and the dumbbells directly under the shoulders.
2. Assume a stance that is substantially wider than the shoulders.
3. Keeping the right leg straight and to the side, squat back and to the left.
4. Lower the hips through a full comfortable range of motion.
5. The left knee can drift slightly in front of the right foot in a line directly over the toes or line up slightly behind the toes depending on what is most comfortable.
6. The back should remain arched, and the head should stay up.
7. Return to the starting position and then repeat in the opposite direction until the desired number of repetitions has been completed.

Common Errors

- Allowing the back to round rather than maintaining an arch.
- Failing to lower the hips through a full comfortable range of motion.
- Allowing the knee of the leg that is supposed to remain straight to bend. (For example, when lowering to the left, the right knee should remain fully extended.)

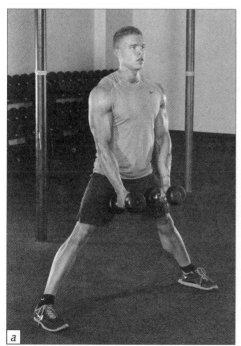
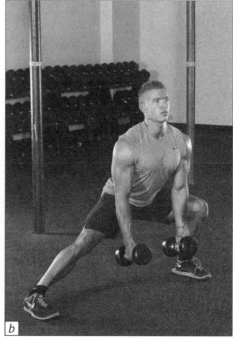

Lunge

Instructions

1. Grasp a dumbbell in each hand, arms at the sides.
2. Assume a shoulder-width stance.
3. Keeping the left leg stationary, step directly forward through an exaggerated range of motion with the right leg.
4. At the forward position the right knee should be over or slightly in front of the right foot, the left leg should be bent and the left knee just off the floor, and the back should be arched and the head up.
5. Return to the starting position with the right leg and repeat the movement with the left leg.

Common Errors

- Allowing the back to round rather than maintaining an arch.
- Failing to take a full stride as you step forward.
- Allowing the knee of the rear leg to touch the floor.
- Taking more than one step to return to the starting position. (To maintain intensity, the feet should return to the starting position in one aggressive step.)

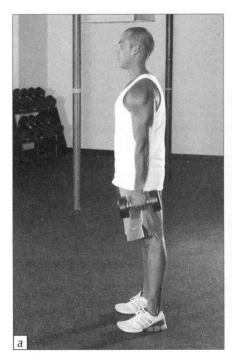
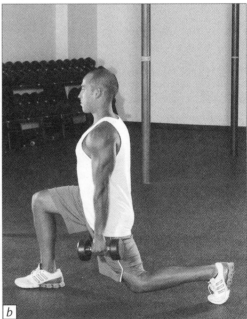

Side Lunge

Instructions

1. Grasp a dumbbell in each hand, with the arms at the sides.
2. Assume a shoulder-width stance.
3. Keeping the right leg straight, take a long step directly to the left.
4. Once you plant your left foot, shift the hips back to achieve a full comfortable depth and range of motion.
5. Keep the back arched and the head up.
6. Return to a shoulder-width stance with one aggressive step.

Common Errors

- Allowing the back to round rather than maintaining an arch in the back.
- Allowing the knee of the "post" leg to bend rather than keeping it fully extended.
- Taking an incomplete recovery step that does not return to the shoulder-width stance before initiating the next lateral step. (One aggressive step should return the lifter to a shoulder-width stance before initiating the next repetition.)

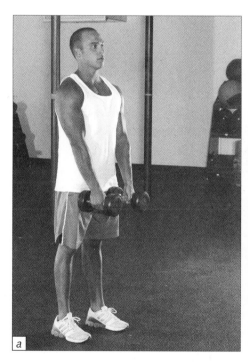

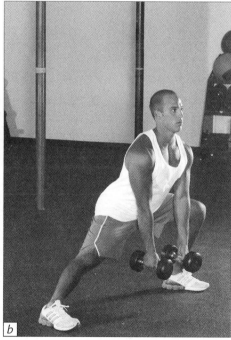

Arc Lunge

Instructions

1. Grasp a dumbbell in each hand with the arms straight at the sides.
2. Assume a shoulder-width stance.
3. Imagine an arc on the floor in front of you. Each point of the arc is a stride length away from you.
4. Divide the arc into sections based on the number of repetitions you will perform.
5. The first repetition will be to the right end of the arc, and the last repetition will be to the left end of the arch. Each step is a progression across the arc, starting at the right end and ending at the left.
6. Keeping the left leg straight, take a long lateral step to the right end of the arc.
7. Once you plant your right foot, shift the hips back to achieve a full comfortable depth and range of motion.
8. Keep the back arched and the head up.
9. Return to a shoulder-width stance with one aggressive step.
10. Alternate stepping with the right and left leg each repetition.
11. The next step will start a gradual progression toward the other end of the arc. With each step you move closer to the center and then across to the opposite end of the arc.
12. Continue until you have completed the required number of repetitions and have progressed from one end of the arc to the other.

Common Errors

- Allowing the back to round rather than maintaining an arch in the back.
- Failing to return to a shoulder-width stance before initiating the next step.
- Failing to progress from one end of the arc to the other with each step.
- Taking a step directly forward to the center of the arch instead taking every step at an angle.
- Failing to move through a full range of motion with every lunge.

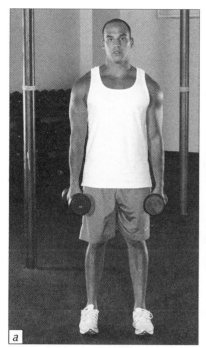

a

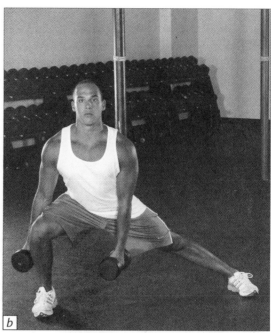

b

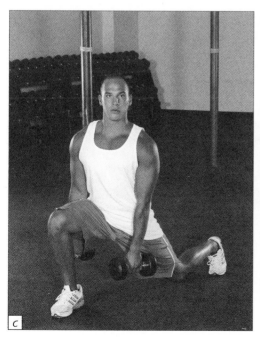

c

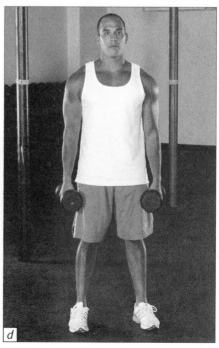

d

Hockey Lunge

Instructions

1. Grasp a dumbbell in each hand with the arms hanging straight at the sides.
2. Assume a shoulder-width stance.
3. Keeping the left leg stationary, step out at a 25- to 30-degree angle that places the foot 18 to 24 inches (46-61 cm) wider than shoulder width (depending on leg length) through an exaggerated range of motion with the right leg.
4. At the forward position, the left knee should be over or slightly in front of the left foot, the right leg should be bent and the right knee just off the floor, and the back should be arched and the head up.
5. Return to the starting position with the right leg and repeat the movement with the right leg, taking that same step 18 to 24 inches wider than shoulder width with the right leg.
6. Return to the starting position in one aggressive step.

Common Errors

- Allowing the back to round rather than maintaining an arch.
- Failing to take a full stride as you step forward at a 25- to 30-degree angle.
- Taking a lateral step that is too narrow.
- Allowing the knee of the rear leg to touch the floor.
- Taking more than one step to return to the starting position.

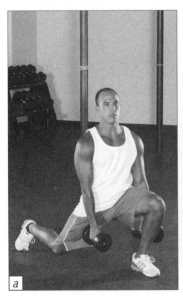
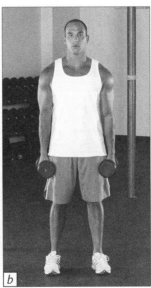
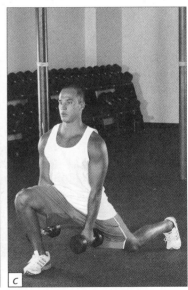

Reverse Lunge

Instructions

1. Grasp a dumbbell in each hand with the arms straight at the sides.
2. Assume a shoulder-width stance.
3. Keeping the left leg stationary, step directly back through an exaggerated range of motion with the right leg.
4. At the back position, the left knee should be over or slightly in front of the left foot, the right leg should be bent and the right knee just off the floor, and the back should be arched and the head up.
5. Take one aggressive step with the right leg to return to the starting position, and repeat the movement with the left leg.

Common Errors

- Allowing the back to round rather than maintaining an arch.
- Failing to take a full stride backward.
- Allowing the knee of the rear leg to touch the floor.
- Taking more than one step to return to the starting position.

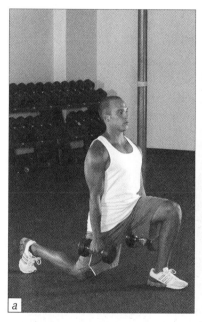
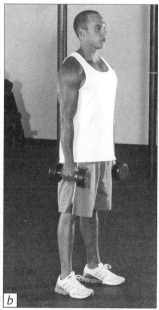
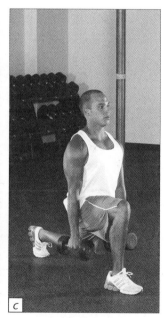

Pivot Lunge

Instructions

1. Grasp a dumbbell in each hand with the arms straight at the sides.
2. Assume a shoulder-width stance.
3. Pivot on the left foot, twisting the body to the right, and lunge to the back and the right of the starting position. If using an imaginary clock to plot the feet, both feet start pointing at 12:00. The right foot moves to a point between 4:00 and 6:00. The body should twist toward the left while stepping behind and to the left with the left foot.
4. At the end position the right knee should be over or slightly in front of the right foot, the left leg should be bent and the left knee just off the floor, and the back should be arched and the head up.
5. Return to a shoulder-width stance with one aggressive step.
6. Repeat in the opposite direction, with the left foot at a spot between 6:00 and 8:00.
7. The angle of the pivot and foot placement can vary on each repetition.

Common Errors

- Allowing the back to round rather than maintaining an arch.
- Failing to take a full stride as you step to the pivot position.
- Allowing the knee of the rear leg to touch the floor.
- Taking more than one step to return to the starting position.

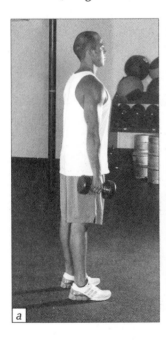
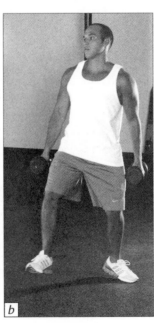
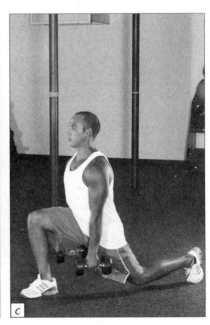

Straight-Leg Deadlift

Instructions

1. Grasp a dumbbell in each hand with the arms fully straightened at the sides.
2. Assume a shoulder-width stance.
3. Lock and then unlock the knees. This is the easiest way to assure the correct start position. Maintain this slightly bent position during the exercise.
4. Arch the back, lift the head, and maintain this position during the exercise.
5. Pivot at the hips and slide the dumbbells down the sides of the legs through a full comfortable range of motion. Range of motion is largely determined by the flexibility of the lower back and hamstrings. Because flexibility differs greatly from person to person, a full and comfortable range of motion is different for each person. Remember to keep the knees straight. The movement occurs at the hips, not the knees.
6. Return to the starting position while maintaining the position of the knees and back.

Common Errors

- Allowing the back to round rather than maintaining an arch.
- Allowing the knees to flex beyond the just-unlocked position.
- Allowing the dumbbells to drift forward as if suspended on a line while lowering them rather than keeping them on the lateral portion of the legs.
- Failing to perform the movement through a complete range of motion.

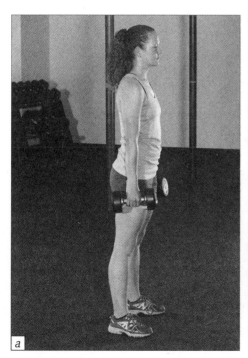
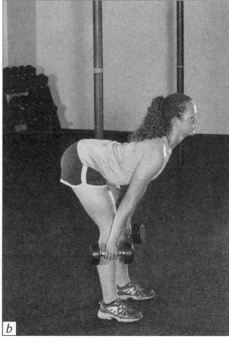

a

b

Calf Raise

Instructions

1. Grasp a dumbbell in the left hand with the left arm hanging straight at the side.
2. Place the left foot on an elevated surface, such as a stair or plyometric box. The surface should be at least 2 inches (5 cm) high. Only the toes and ball of the right foot are in contact with the surface.
3. Bend the right leg at the knee to elevate the right foot off the floor. It should remain elevated without contacting the floor during performance of the exercise.
4. Hold onto something stable with the right hand. Use the right arm only for balance. It should not assist in performance of the movement.
5. Using the muscles of the left foot only, elevate onto the toes as high as you can.
6. Lower the left foot so that the heel of the foot drops below the surface you are standing on.
7. Lift and lower under control. Once the required repetitions have been completed, repeat the exercise on the right foot.

Common Errors

- Failing to achieve a full range of motion, either not going as high as possible or as low as possible.
- Using the support arm to assist in the movement rather than only for balance.
- Performing the movement too quickly and using momentum to help perform the exercise. (Both the lifting and lowering phase should be controlled.)

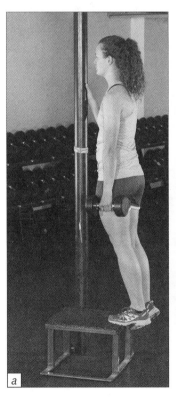
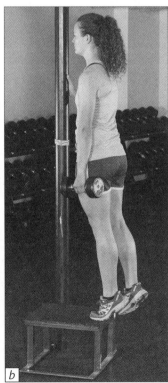
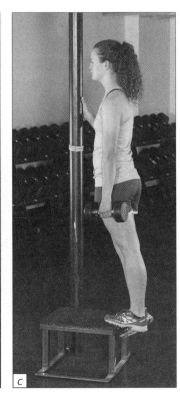

Step-Up

Instructions

1. Grasp a dumbbell in each hand with the arms straight at the sides.

2. Stand behind a plyometric box or exercise bench with your left foot on it. This surface should be high enough that your left knee is 1 to 2 inches (2.5-5 cm) higher than the right hip.

3. Using the muscles of the left leg, elevate the body and place the left foot in a shoulder-width stance next to the left foot.

4. Keep the left foot in place and step down with the right foot. You are now in a shoulder-width stance with the right foot elevated and the left foot on the floor.

5. Continue alternating stepping up with each leg until you have completed the required number of repetitions.

Common Errors

• Using the leg on the floor to help elevate the body. (Only the leg on the bench should be used to lift the body.)

• Rounding the back or bending forward at the trunk rather than maintaining an upright position.

• Failure to lift and lower the body under control.

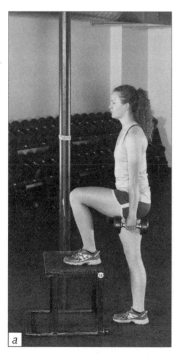
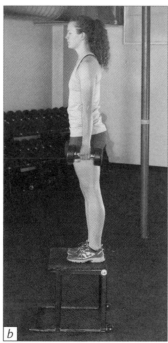
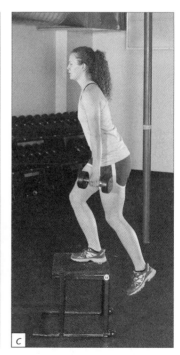

a

b

c

CHAPTER 6

Core

Many people associate training the core with improved aesthetics and want to improve their appearance by developing flat "six-pack" abs. For people training for general fitness or improved appearance, this is a reasonable goal. For athletes, however, core training is much more about enhancing physical performance than improving appearance. Because the core plays an important role in many sports, improving core strength and power can enhance athletic performance.

Despite the fact that most people associate core training with strengthening the abs, the core also includes the muscles of the lower back. A strong lower back, in conjunction with strong abdominals, is important for optimal performance in most athletic activities (e.g., swinging a bat, tackling, running, jumping). Further, a strong core helps transfer forces developed in the lower body through the midsection and to the upper body in activities such as throwing, hitting, jerking a barbell or dumbbell, and blocking.

Increases in strength occur as a result of providing overload and progression during training. Unfortunately, many people make the mistake of attempting to strengthen the core by using low-intensity, high-repetition training, such as one set of 100. While the core is predominately made up of Type I (slow-twitch) endurance fibers (because of the need to support the trunk in an upright position), higher-intensity training is still required to bring about maximal increases in strength in the core. All of the exercises presented here use dumbbells to overload the musculature. The typical repetition range for the exercises is 8 to 25, and the resistance should be high enough to be challenging for the number of repetitions performed. One would not perform one set of 100 squats to get stronger; the same is true when training the core.

ABDOMINALS

The primary abdominal muscles are the rectus abdominis, obliques, and transverse abdominis.

Crunch

Instructions

1. Lie faceup on the floor, bend the knees, and place the soles of the feet flat on the floor.
2. Holding both ends of the dumbbell, turn it sideways so it is lying across the upper chest.
3. Keeping the dumbbell high on the upper chest, crunch straight up as if trying to touch the chin to the ceiling. Elevate the upper back off the floor as high as possible while maintaining correct technique. Remember that this is a crunch and not a sit-up. There should be no flexion of the spine. Remember to emphasize lifting the head and chest straight up towards the ceiling.
4. As you lower, touch the upper back to the floor before starting the next repetition.
5. Try to set a pace of two seconds up and two seconds down.

Common Errors

- Allowing the dumbbell to roll down the chest as you crunch. (The position of the dumbbell should be constant during the exercise.)
- Pointing the chin toward the wall rather than elevating it toward the ceiling during the crunch. (The crunching motion should be straight up.)
- Pausing in the low position with the upper back resting on the floor between repetitions.
- Failing to move through the full range of motion.

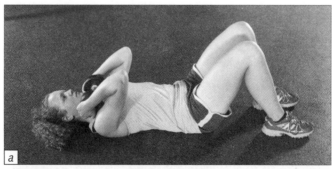

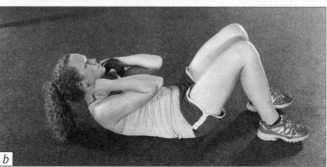

Decline Crunch

Instructions

1. Lie on your back on a decline bench. Start with a decline of 15 degrees and gradually increase the degree as you build strength, making sure to maintain correct technique when increasing the degree of decline used.
2. Bend the knees and place the legs through the pads or rollers to secure yourself on the bench.
3. Holding both ends of a dumbbell, turn it sideways so it is lying across the upper chest.
4. Keeping the dumbbell high on the upper chest, crunch straight up as if trying to touch the chin to the ceiling. Remember this is a crunch and not a sit-up.

Common Errors

- Allowing the dumbbell to roll down the chest as you crunch rather than holding it in place.
- Pointing the chin toward the wall rather than elevating it toward the ceiling during the crunch. (The crunching motion should be straight up.)
- Pausing in the low position with the upper back resting on the floor between repetitions.
- Failing to move through a full range of motion and elevating the chin toward the ceiling as high as possible.

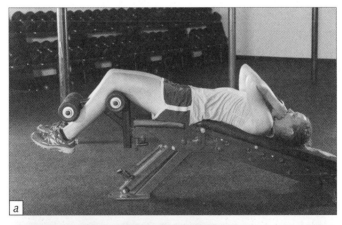

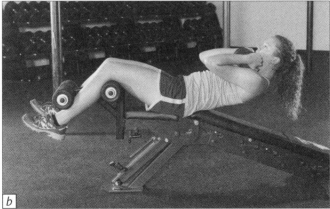

Twisting Crunch

Instructions

1. Lie faceup on the floor.
2. Holding both ends of a dumbbell, turn it sideways across the upper chest.
3. Keeping the dumbbell high on the chest, crunch up and twist simultaneously as if trying to touch the right shoulder to the ceiling.
4. Elevate the chin and shoulder toward the ceiling as high as possible while remembering this is a crunch and not a sit-up.
5. Lower to the start position and repeat the movement in the opposite direction.

Common Errors

- Allowing the dumbbell to roll down the chest as you crunch rather than holding the dumbbell steady.
- Crunching in a motion that lifts the chin toward the wall rather than the ceiling.
- Failing to crunch straight up and twist simultaneously.
- Pausing in the low position and resting the upper back on the floor between repetitions.
- Failing to move through the full range of motion.

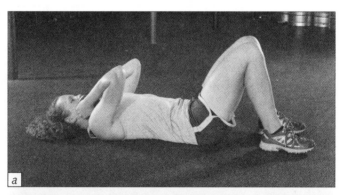

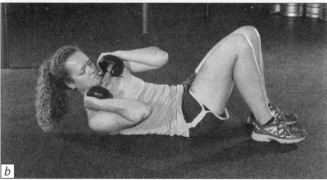

Decline Twisting Crunch

Instructions

1. Lie faceup on a decline bench. Start with a decline of 15 degrees. The degree of decline can be increased gradually to 30 degrees or more.
2. Bend the knees and place the legs through the pads or rollers to secure yourself on the bench.
3. Holding both ends of the dumbbell, turn it sideways across the upper chest. Keeping the dumbbell high on the upper chest, crunch up and twist simultaneously as if trying to touch the right shoulder to the ceiling.

Common Errors

- Allowing the dumbbell to roll down the chest as you crunch rather than holding the dumbbell steady.
- Crunching in a motion that lifts the chin toward the wall rather than the ceiling.
- Failing to crunch straight up and twist simultaneously.
- Pausing in the low position and resting the upper back on the floor between repetitions.
- Failing to move through the full range of motion.

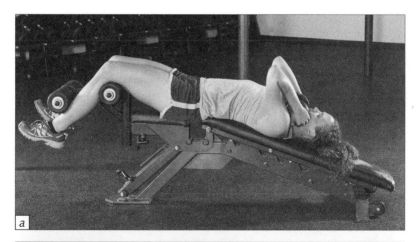

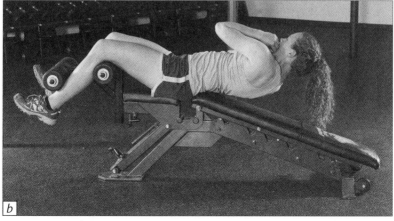

Toe Touch

Instructions

1. Lie face up on the floor.
2. Turn a dumbbell on end and grasp the inside edge of its top end.
3. Fully extend the arms to press the dumbbell up directly above the face.
4. Keeping the legs straight, lift them until they are nearly at a 90-degree angle.
5. Crunch up, bringing the dumbbell up toward the toes. The ability to touch the dumbbell to the toes depends on limb length and flexibility.
6. Lower until the upper back touches the floor and then immediately repeat the movement; there should be no pause in the bottom position.

Common Errors

- Not fully straightening knees.
- Positioning the feet directly over the hips. (The feet should be 4 to 6 inches [10-15 cm] short of being directly over the hips.)
- Pausing at the bottom of the movement and resting the back on the floor.
- Failing to crunch up through the full range of motion.

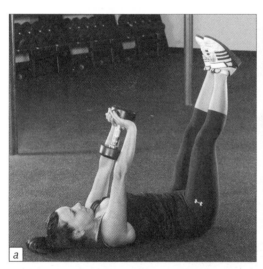
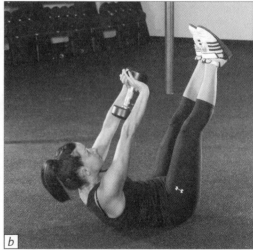

Alternating Toe Touch

Instructions

1. Lie faceup on the floor.
2. Turn a dumbbell on end and securely grasp the inside edge of its top end.
3. Fully extend the arms to press the dumbbell up over the chest.
4. With the legs fully extended, lift them until the feet are 4 to 6 inches (10-15 cm) short of being directly over the hips.
5. Crunch up and twist, bringing the dumbbell up toward outside of the left leg.
6. Lower until the upper back touches the floor and then immediately repeat the movement; there should be no pause in the bottom position.
7. Repeat on the other side, bringing the dumbbell up toward the outside of the right leg.
8. The ability to touch the dumbbell to the toes depends on limb length and flexibility.

Common Errors

- Failing to keep the legs straight.
- Positioning the feet directly over the hips rather than raising the legs just short of a 90-degree angle.
- Pausing at the bottom of the movement and resting the back on the floor.
- Failing to crunch up through the full range of motion.
- Failing to twist enough that the dumbbell touches the outside of the leg on each repetition.

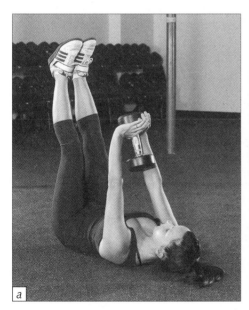
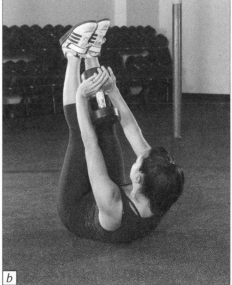

V-Up

Instructions

1. Lie faceup on the floor and fully extend the legs.
2. Grasp the inside edge of the top the dumbbell.
3. Fully extend the arms behind the head, keeping the bottom of the dumbbell on the floor.
4. Keeping the arms and legs straight, lift them simultaneously until the dumbbell touches, or nearly touches, the legs.
5. Lower until the upper back touches the floor and then immediately repeat the movement; there should be no pause in the bottom position.

Common Errors

- Failing to keep the arms and legs straight.
- Not crunching as high as possible. (The dumbbell should touch the legs as close to the feet as possible.)
- Pausing at the bottom of the movement and resting the back on the floor.

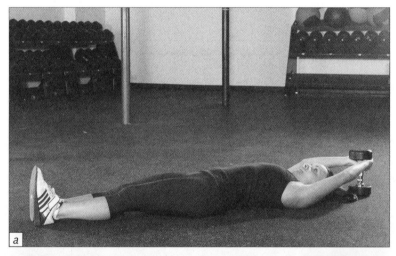

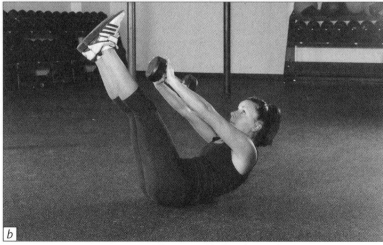

Alternating V-Up

Instructions

1. Lie faceup on the floor and fully extend the legs.
2. Grasp the inside edge of the top of the dumbbell and fully extend the arms behind the head, keeping the bottom of the dumbbell on the floor.
3. Keeping the arms and legs straight, simultaneously lift them while twisting the trunk to touch the dumbbell to the outside of the left leg.
4. The legs should be raised until they are just short of a 90-degree angle.
5. Simultaneously lower the legs and upper back to the floor before initiating the next repetition.
6. Lower until the upper back touches the floor and then immediately repeat the movement; there should be no pause in the bottom position.
7. Repeat, bringing the dumbbell to the outside of the right leg.

Common Errors

- Failing to keep the arms and legs straight.
- Not crunching as high as possible. (The dumbbell should touch the legs as close to the feet as possible.)
- Pausing at the bottom of the movement and resting the back on the floor.

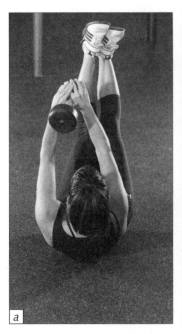 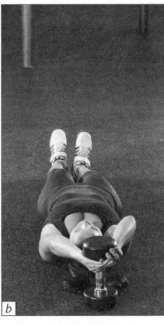 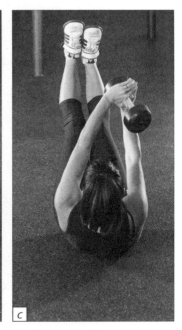

Press Crunch

Instructions

1. Lie faceup with knees bent and feet flat on the floor.
2. Turn a dumbbell on end and grasp the inside edge of the top.
3. Straighten the arms and press the dumbbell up over the chest.
4. Crunch up, pressing the dumbbell toward the ceiling.
5. Lower until the upper back touches the floor and then immediately repeat the movement; there should be no pause in the bottom position.

Common Errors

- Failing to fully extend the arms.
- Pausing at the bottom of the movement and resting the back on the floor.
- Not crunching up through the full range of motion.

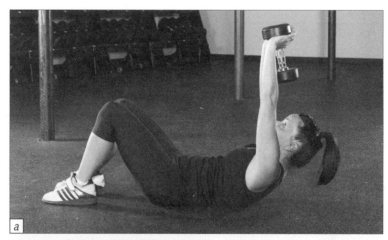

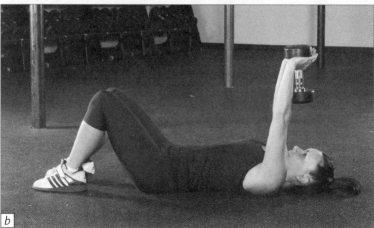

Decline Press Crunch

Instructions

1. Lie faceup on a decline bench. Start with a decline of 15 degrees. Gradually increase the degree of the decline as you build core strength.
2. Bend the knees and place the legs through the pads or rollers to secure yourself.
3. Grasp the inside edge of the top of the dumbbell and straighten the arms to press the dumbbell over the chest.
4. Crunch up, pressing the dumbbell toward the ceiling.
5. Lower until the upper back touches the bench and then immediately repeat the movement; there should be no pause in the bottom position.

Common Errors

- Not fully extending the arms.
- Pausing at the bottom of the movement and resting the back on the bench.
- Failing to crunch through the full range of motion.

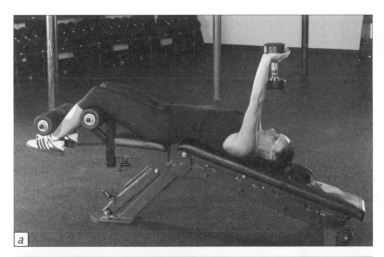

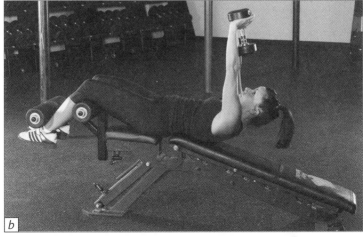

Alternating Press Crunch

Instructions

1. Lie faceup and bend the knees so the feet are flat on the floor.
2. Grasp the inside edge of the top of the dumbbell and straighten the arms to press the dumbbell over the chest.
3. Crunch up, pressing the dumbbell toward the ceiling and the outside of the right leg.
4. Repeat the movement, pressing the dumbbell toward the ceiling and the outside of the left leg.
5. Lower until the upper back touches the floor and then immediately repeat the movement; there should be no pause in the bottom position.

Common Errors

- Not fully extending the arms.
- Pausing at the bottom of the movement, resting the back on the floor.
- Failing to crunch through the full range of motion.
- Not touching the dumbbell to the outside of the leg.

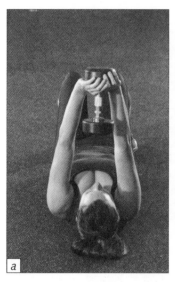
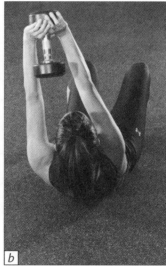
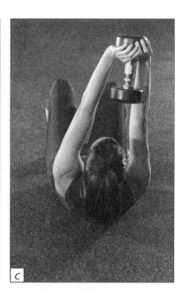

Decline Alternating Press Crunch

Instructions

1. Lie faceup on a decline bench. Start with a decline of 15 degrees. Gradually increase the degree of the decline as you build core strength.
2. Bend the knees and place the legs through the pads or rollers to secure yourself.
3. Grasp the inside edge of the top of the dumbbell and straighten the arms to press the dumbbell over the chest.
4. Crunch up, pressing the dumbbell toward the ceiling and the outside of the left leg.
5. Lower until the upper back touches the floor and then immediately repeat the movement; there should be no pause in the bottom position.
6. Repeat the movement, this time pressing the dumbbell toward the ceiling and the outside of the right leg.

Common Errors

- Not fully extending the arms.
- Pausing at the bottom of the movement and resting the back on the bench.
- Failing to crunch up through the full range of motion.
- Not touching the dumbbell to the outside of the leg.

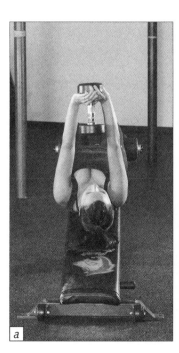
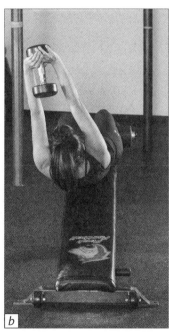
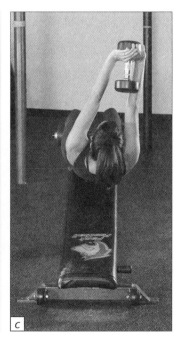

LOWER BACK

The primary lower back muscles are the erector spinae, obliques, gluteus maximus, and adductor magnus.

Back Extension

Instructions

1. Position yourself on a back extension bench. You can also use an incline bench by lying facedown so that the body from the waist up is hanging off the bench. A partner anchors your legs to the bench.
2. Hold a dumbbell sideways across your upper chest.
3. Start in the bottom position bent at the waist so that the head is near the floor and the shoulders are nearly directly under the hips.
4. Keeping the back flat and flexing at the hip, lift the trunk without using momentum.
5. When using a back extension bench, the trunk should be lifted until the center of the shoulder joint is at the same height as the center of the hip joint.
6. When performing the movement on an incline bench, the trunk should be lifted until the center of the shoulder joint is in a straight line with the center of the hip, knee, and ankle joints.
7. Lower the trunk under control until the shoulder joints are directly under the hip joints. You should attempt to lower the head as close to the floor as possible while keeping the back flat.

Common Errors

- Not fully lowering to the bottom position.
- Failing to achieve the desired height at the top of the movement. (The shoulder joint should be in a straight line with the hip joint. The top of the lift should stop with this straight-line position and no higher.)
- Using momentum to assist in lifting the trunk.
- Failing to control the rate of descent.

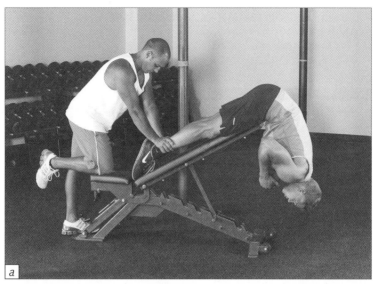

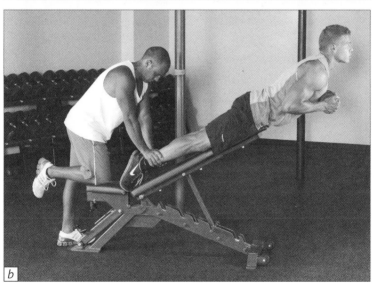

Twisting Back Extension

Instructions

1. Place yourself on a back extension bench. You can also use an incline bench by lying facedown so that the body from the waist up is hanging off the bench. A partner anchors your legs to the bench.
2. Hold a dumbbell sideways across your upper chest.
3. Start in the bottom position bent at the waist so that the head is near the floor and the shoulders are nearly directly under the hips.
4. Keeping the back flat and without using momentum, flex at the hip and simultaneously lift and twist the trunk so that at the top position the right shoulder points toward the ceiling.
5. Controlling the descent, slowly lower the body to the starting position.
6. Repeat the movement, twisting in the opposite direction.
7. When using a back extension bench, lift the trunk until the center of the shoulder joint is at the same height as the center of the hip joint.
8. When performing the movement on an incline bench, lift the trunk until the center of the shoulder joint is in a straight line with the center of the hip, knee, and ankle joints.

Common Errors

- Not fully lowering to the bottom position.
- Rising too high or not high enough at the top of the movement. (The shoulder joint should be in a straight line with the hip joint. Achieve this straight-line position and no higher.)
- Using momentum to assist in lifting the trunk.
- Not controlling the rate of descent.

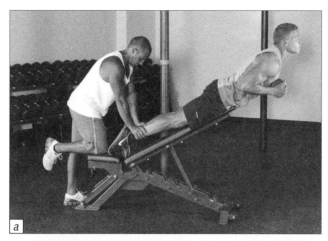

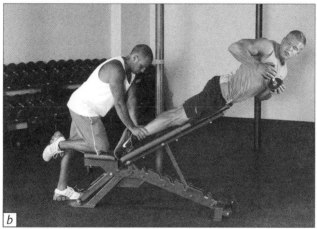

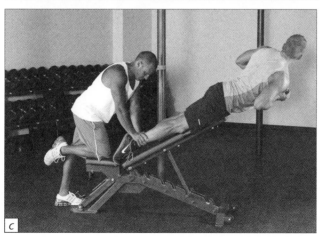

CHAPTER 7

Total Body

Total-body exercises, those using the major muscles groups in both the lower and upper body, are the weightlifting movements, better known as Olympic lifts. The weightlifting movements consist of cleans, jerks, and snatches plus all of their associated training exercises.

These total-body exercises have significant advantages over other types of exercises when performed with dumbbells. Most importantly, they are performed explosively. Lifters attempt to accelerate the weight as quickly as possible. The weightlifting movements result in high power outputs because of this acceleration phase. Research has shown that the power resulting from the weightlifting movements is significantly greater than the power that results from more traditional movements, such as the bench, squat, or deadlift. In most sports, the limiting factor in optimal performance is the ability to generate power not strength levels. Further, when using dumbbells, the variety of exercises is increased because dumbbell training allows both alternating and single arm movements, which obviously can't be performed with a barbell.

Although it is beyond the scope of this book, another training method that increases power is plyometric training. In chapter 9, Training for Increased Power, plyometric exercises are part of the training regimen. Plyometric training uses a variety of exercises that take advantage of the stretch-shortening cycle that occurs when a muscle is stretched. This stretch-shortening cycle results in a more explosive muscular contraction.

It is possible to combine the exercises in this chapter and in previous chapters. For example, you could perform a power clean to a power jerk, or a front squat to a split alternating-foot jerk. The combinations are endless and only limited by your creativity. One of the primary advantages to combining these lifts is their positive effect on muscular endurance. And performing combination lifts during a hypertrophy cycle is beneficial because of the additional muscle mass recruited during each repetition.

One note of explanation is needed here. In many of the exercise descriptions below you will see the phrases *catch the dumbbells* or *catch the dumbbell*. The dumbbells are not literally leaving the hands so that they have to be caught. However, in many of the exercises, the dumbbells will be moving at a high rate of speed. To catch the dumbbell means that the dumbbells are brought to a complete stop under control and in good position.

Push Press

Instructions

1. Stand with the feet about shoulder-width apart and rest a pair of dumbbells on the shoulders.
2. Sit back at the hips to the depth you would normally achieve when performing a vertical-jump attempt. Keep the heels on the floor.
3. At the bottom of the jump action, quickly rise and transfer the momentum by pushing against the ground through the lower body and core to the upper body. This momentum will cause the dumbbells to lift off the shoulders slightly.
4. When the dumbbells have lifted off the shoulders, fully extend the arms to press the dumbbells straight up over the shoulders.
5. Pause in this position for a second and then lower the dumbbells to the starting position.

Common Errors

- Placing the feet either wider or narrower than shoulder width.
- Initiating the movement by flexing the knees forward rather than flexing the hips back.
- Pausing at the bottom of the exercise rather than changing direction as quickly as possible.
- Pressing the dumbbells off the shoulders too soon rather than waiting until they have risen off the shoulders as a result of the action in the lower body.
- Pressing the dumbbells too quickly. (The movement is no faster than in a dumbbell shoulder press.)
- Not pausing at the top of the movement for a second to demonstrate control before lowering the dumbbells.

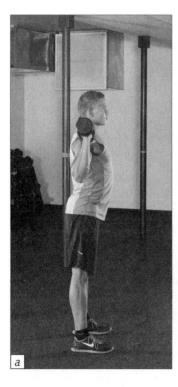
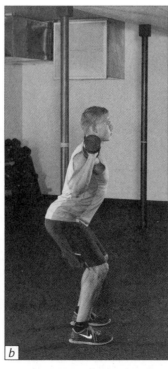
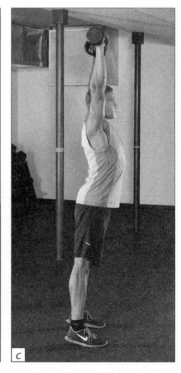

Alternating Push Press

Instructions

1. Stand with the feet about shoulder-width apart and rest a pair of dumbbells on the shoulders.
2. Sit back until you are at the depth of a vertical-jump attempt. Keep the heels on the floor.
3. At the bottom of the jump action, quickly rise and transfer the momentum by pushing against the ground through the lower body and core to the upper body.
4. This momentum will cause the dumbbells to lift off the shoulders slightly.
5. When the dumbbells have risen off the shoulder, fully extend the right arm to press the dumbbell over the right shoulder.
6. Pause in this position for a second, and then lower the dumbbell in the right arm back to the starting position.
7. Repeat the movement, performing the movement with the left arm.

Common Errors

- Placing the feet either wider or narrower than shoulder width.
- Starting the movement by flexing the knees forward rather than flexing the hips back.
- Pausing at the bottom of the motion rather than changing direction as quickly as possible.
- Pressing the dumbbell over the shoulder before it has risen off the shoulder as a result of the action in the lower body.
- Pressing the dumbbell too quickly. (The movement is no faster than when performing a dumbbell shoulder press.)
- Not pausing at the top of the movement for a second to demonstrate control before lowering the dumbbell.

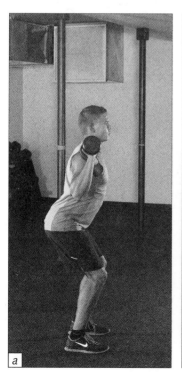
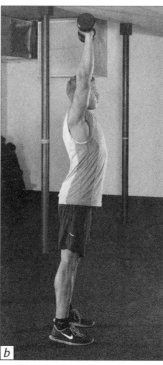
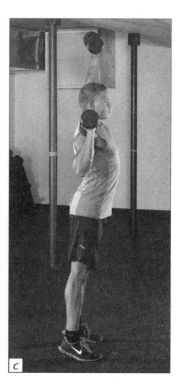

a   b   c

One-Arm Push Press

Instructions

1. Stand with the feet about shoulder width apart.
2. Grasp a dumbbell in the right hand and rest it on the right shoulder.
3. Sit back until you are at the depth of a vertical-jump attempt. Keep the heels on the floor.
4. At the bottom of the jump action, quickly rise and transfer the momentum by pushing against the ground through the lower body and core to the upper body.
5. This momentum will cause the dumbbell to lift off the shoulder slightly. At this point fully extend the right arm to press the dumbbell over the right shoulder.
6. Pause in this position for a second and then lower the dumbbell to the starting position.
7. Complete the required number of repetitions and then repeat the exercise with the left arm.

Common Errors

- Placing the feet either wider or narrow than shoulder width.
- Initiating the movement by flexing the knees forward rather than flexing the hips back.
- Pausing at the bottom of the jump position rather than changing direction as quickly as possible.
- Pressing the dumbbell over the shoulder before it has risen off the shoulders as a result of the action in the lower body.
- Pressing the dumbbell too quickly. (The movement is no faster than when performing a dumbbell shoulder press.)
- Not pausing at the top of the movement for a second to demonstrate control before lowering the dumbbell.

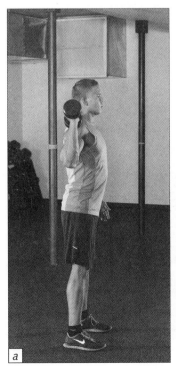
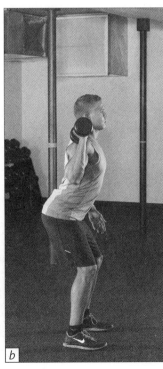
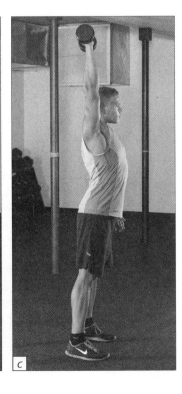

a   b   c

Power Jerk

Instructions

1. Stand with the feet about shoulder-width apart and rest a pair of dumbbells on the shoulders.
2. Sit back until you are at the depth of a vertical-jump attempt. Keep the heels on the floor.
3. At the bottom of the jump action, quickly rise and transfer the momentum by pushing against the ground through the lower body and core to the upper body.
4. The force generated in the lower body should cause the dumbbells to lift off of the shoulders. At this point, quickly extend the arms until they are straight and the dumbbells are directly over the shoulders. The arms steer the dumbbells to the correct position. Very little pressing action should be involved.
5. Pause in this position for a second and then lower the dumbbells to the starting position.

Common Errors

- Placing the feet either wider or narrower than shoulder width.
- Initiating the movement by flexing the knees forward rather than flexing the hips back.
- Pausing at the bottom of the jump position rather than changing direction as quickly as possible.
- Using the arms too soon to press the dumbbells off the shoulders.
- Pressing the dumbbells too quickly. (The movement is no faster than when performing a dumbbell shoulder press.)
- Not pausing at the top of the movement for a second to demonstrate control before lowering the dumbbells.

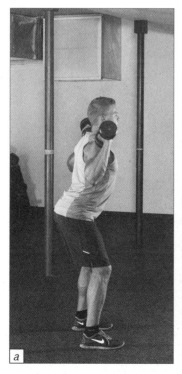 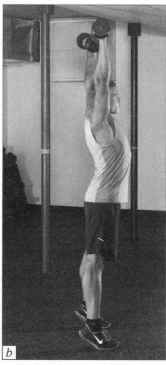

Alternating Power Jerk

Instructions

1. Stand with the feet shoulder-width apart and rest a pair of dumbbells on the shoulders.
2. Sit back until you are at the depth of a vertical-jump attempt. Keep the heels on the floor.
3. At the bottom of the jump action, quickly rise up and transfer the momentum by pushing against the ground through the lower body and core to the upper body.
4. The force generated in the lower body should lift the dumbbells off of the shoulders. At this point, quickly extend the left arm until it is straight and the dumbbell is directly over the right shoulder. The arm steers the dumbbell to the correct position. Very little pressing action should be involved.
5. Pause in this position for a second and then lower the dumbbell to the starting position.
6. Repeat the movement with the right arm.

Common Errors

- Placing the feet either wider or narrower than shoulder width.
- Initiating the movement by flexing the knees forward rather than flexing the hips back.
- Pausing at the bottom of the jump position rather than changing direction as quickly as possible.
- Using the arms before the dumbbells have risen off the shoulders as a result of the action in the lower body.
- Lifting the dumbbells with the arms instead of letting the lower-body momentum lift them.
- Not pausing at the top of the movement for a second to demonstrate control before lowering the dumbbell.

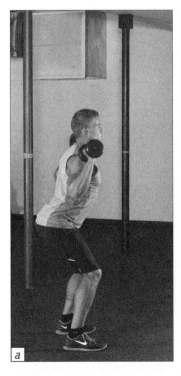 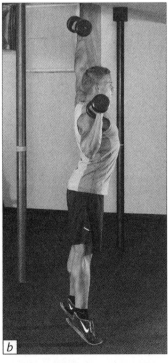

One-Arm Power Jerk

Instructions

1. Stand with the feet about shoulder-width apart and hold a dumbbell in the right hand, resting it on the right shoulder.
2. Sit back until you are at the depth of a vertical-jump attempt. Keep the heels on the floor.
3. At the bottom of the jump action, quickly rise and transfer the momentum by pushing against the ground through the lower body and core to the upper body.
4. This momentum will cause the dumbbell to quickly lift off the shoulder. Continue raising the dumbbell until the right arm is fully extended. The right arm steers the dumbbell to the correct position. Very little pressing action should be involved.
5. Pause in this position for a second and then lower the dumbbell back to the starting position.
6. Complete the required number of repetitions and then repeat the exercise with the left arm.

Common Errors

- Placing the feet either wider or narrower than shoulder width.
- Initiating the movement by flexing the knees forward rather than flexing the hips back.
- Pausing at the bottom of the jump position instead of changing direction as quickly as possible.
- Using the arm too soon to press the dumbbell off the shoulder. (The arm should not come into play until the dumbbell has risen off the shoulders as a result of the action in the lower body.)
- Using the arm to lift before the dumbbell has risen off the shoulder as a result of the action in the lower body.
- Not pausing at the top of the movement for a second to demonstrate control before lowering the dumbbell.

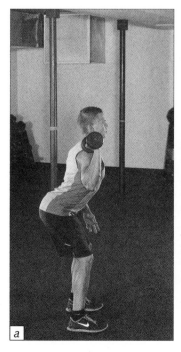
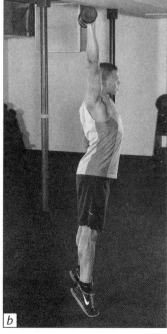

a

b

Split Alternating-Feet Jerk

Instructions

1. Stand with the feet about shoulder-width apart and rest a pair of dumbbells on the shoulders.
2. Sit back until you are at the depth of a vertical-jump attempt. Keep the heels on the floor.
3. At the bottom of the jump action, quickly rise and transfer the momentum by pushing against the ground through the lower body and core to the upper body.
4. The force generated in the lower body should cause the dumbbells to quickly lift off of the shoulders.
5. When the hips are fully extended, quickly split the feet, with the left foot moving forward and the right foot moving back so you catch the dumbbells in what could be called a slight lunge position.
6. While splitting under the dumbbells, continue to press them until the elbows are fully extended and locked. The arms steer the dumbbells to the correct position. Very little pressing should be involved.
7. Return the feet to the starting position by stepping up with the right foot and stepping back with the left foot.
8. Pause in this position for a second and then lower the dumbbells to the starting position.
9. Alternate the split position each repetition.

Common Errors

- Placing the feet either wider or narrower than shoulder width.
- Initiating the movement by flexing the knees forward rather than flexing the hips back.
- Pausing at the bottom of the jump position instead of changing direction as quickly as possible.
- Using the arms to lift the dumbbells off the shoulders instead of using them only to steer the dumbbells to the correct catch position.
- Lowering the dumbbells before the feet are fully recovered to the start position.

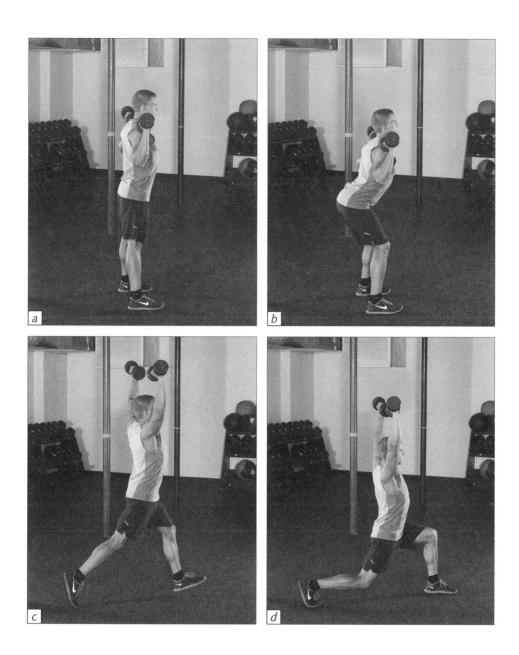

Split Alternating-Feet Alternating-Arm Jerk

Instructions

1. Stand with the feet about shoulder-width apart and rest a pair of dumbbells on the shoulders.
2. Sit back until you are at the depth of a vertical-jump attempt. Keep the heels on the floor.
3. At the bottom of the jump action, quickly rise and transfer the momentum by pushing against the ground through the lower body and core to the upper body.
4. The force generated in the lower body should cause the dumbbells to quickly lift off of the shoulders.
5. When the hips are fully extended, quickly split the feet, with the left foot moving forward and the right foot moving back so you catch the dumbbells in what could be called a high lunge position.
6. While splitting under the dumbbell, continue to lift the dumbbell in the right hand until the elbow is fully extended and locked. The arm steers the dumbbell to the correct position. Very little pressing action should be involved.
7. Return the feet to the starting position, stepping up with the right foot and stepping back with the left foot.
8. Pause in this position for a second and then lower the dumbbell back to the starting position.
9. Alternate the split position and the arm assisting the lift of dumbbell each repetition.
10. In the top position the arm that has been raised will always be on the opposite side of the leg that has moved forward (e.g., right leg forward, left arm up).

Common Errors

- Placing the feet either wider or narrower than shoulder width.
- Initiating the movement by flexing the knees forward rather than flexing the hips back.
- Pausing at the bottom of the jump position instead of changing direction as quickly as possible.
- Using the arms to press the dumbbells off the shoulders instead of to steer the dumbbells to the correct catch position.
- Lowering the dumbbells before the feet are fully recovered to the start position.
- Lifting the arm on the same side as the forward leg.

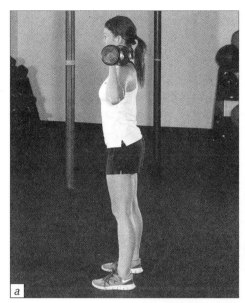

a

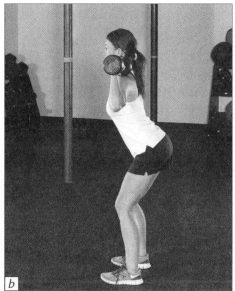

b

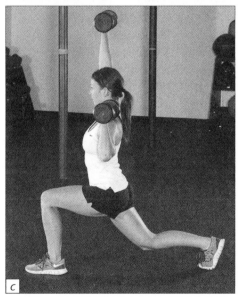

c

Split Alternating-Feet One-Arm Jerk

Instructions

1. Stand with the feet about shoulder-width apart and rest a dumbbell on the right shoulder.
2. Sit back until you are at the depth of a vertical-jump attempt. Keep the heels on the floor.
3. At the bottom of the jump action, quickly rise and transfer the momentum by pushing against the ground through the lower body and core to the upper body.
4. The force generated in the lower body should cause the dumbbell to quickly lift off of the shoulder.
5. When the hips are fully extended, quickly split the feet, with the left foot moving forward and the right foot moving back so you catch the dumbbells in what could be called a high lunge position.
6. While splitting under the dumbbell continue to press it until the elbow is fully extended and locked. The arm mainly steers the dumbbell to the correct position. Very little pressing action should be involved.
7. Pause in this position for a second, recover the feet to the start position by stepping up with the left foot and back with the right foot to bring them together, and then lower the dumbbell to the starting position.
8. Alternate the split position with each repetition while completing the full number of repetitions on the right arm.
9. Once you have completed the repetition on the right arm, switch the dumbbell to the left hand.

Common Errors

- Placing the feet either wider or narrower than shoulder width.
- Initiating the movement by flexing the knees forward rather than flexing the hips back.
- Pausing at the bottom of the jump position instead of changing direction as quickly as possible.
- Using the arm to press the dumbbell off the shoulder instead of to steer the dumbbell to the correct catch position.
- Lowering the dumbbell before the feet are fully recovered to the start position.
- Lifting the arm on the same side as the forward leg.

Note: All of the following dumbbell clean and dumbbell snatch exercises can be performed from both a hang position as well as performing the full movement. The full movements are performed with a start position holding the dumbbells at approximately mid-shin height, or replicating the position achieved when performing the movement with a barbell and full-sized weight plates positioned on the bar. Otherwise, the movement from the hang position and from mid-shin are both very similar.

Because the mid-shin start position involves a greater range of motion in which to perform the exercise, typically more weight can be used from this lower start position. However, the hang start position typically is easier to learn than the full movement, so the recommendation is to learn the movement using the hang position and then, once that movement has been perfected, move to the mid-shin start position.

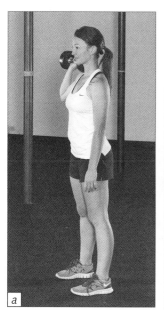
a

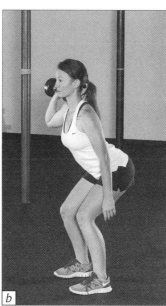
b

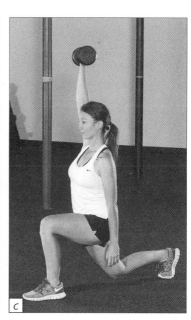
c

Hang Power Clean

Instructions

1. Stand with the feet about shoulder-width apart.

2. With the arms hanging at the sides, hold a pair of dumbbells at the sides of the legs.

3. Sit back at the hips, keeping the back arched and the head up, and lower the dumbbells until the handles are positioned at the desired start position height (i.e., with the handle of the dumbbell centered with the knee joint when performing from the hang start position, and from mid-shin when performing the full movement).

4. The shoulders should be slightly in front of the dumbbells. If the shoulders are not in front of the knees, straighten the knees until achieving this position.

5. To begin the lift, push against the ground to extend the hip, knee, and ankle joints.

6. After achieving full extension, aggressively shrug the shoulders to elevate the dumbbells slightly.

7. Once the shrug is complete, pull the dumbbells along the rib cage to the lower portion of the armpits.

8. From this position, pull the body under the dumbbells by flexing at the hips and aggressively bringing the elbows around to rack the back half of the dumbbells on the shoulders while catching the dumbbells in a quarter-squat position.

9. In this racked position, the head should be up and the back arched, the elbows should be high, and the knees should be behind the toes.

10. Once the dumbbells are on the shoulders, extend the knees and hips so you are in a fully upright position.

Common Errors

- Placing the feet either wider or narrower than shoulder width.
- Holding the dumbbells either above or below the knee joint.
- In the start position, placing the shoulders either over or behind the dumbbells instead of slightly in front of them.
- Bending the elbows before the ankles, knees, and hips are fully extended and the shoulders are at the top of the shrug.
- Bringing the dumbbells to the shoulders in an arched movement rather than straight up to the armpits.
- Sitting under the dumbbells by flexing at the knees and bringing them in front of the toes instead of by sitting back at the hips.
- Catching with the elbows pointing toward the floor rather than toward the wall.
- Sitting too deep in the catching action rather than just deep enough to rack the dumbbells on the shoulders.

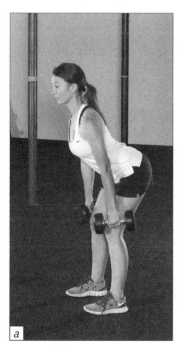 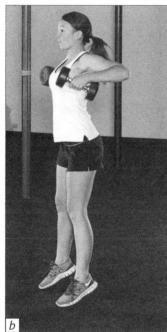 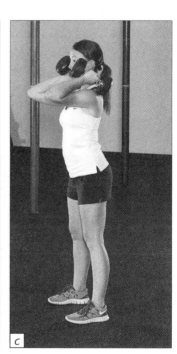

Alternating Power Clean

Instructions

1. Stand with the feet about shoulder-width apart.
2. With the arms hanging at the sides, hold a pair of dumbbells at the sides of the legs.
3. Sit back at the hips, keep the back arched and the head up, and lower the dumbbells until the handles of the dumbbells are positioned at the desired start position height (i.e., with the handle of the dumbbell centered with the knee joint when performing from the hang start position, and from mid-shin when performing the full movement).
4. The shoulders should be slightly in front of the dumbbells. If the shoulders are not in front of the knees, straighten the knees until achieving this position.
5. To begin the lift, push against the ground to extend the hip, knee, and ankle joints.
6. After achieving full extension, aggressively shrug the shoulders to elevate the dumbbells slightly.
7. Once the shrug is complete, pull the dumbbell in the left hand along the rib cage to the lower portion of the armpit.
8. From this position pull the body under the dumbbell by flexing at the hips and aggressively bringing the right elbow around to rack the back half of the dumbbell on the left shoulder while catching the dumbbells in a quarter-squat position.
9. In this racked position, the head should be up and the back arched, the elbow should be high, and the knees should be behind the toes.
10. Once the dumbbell has been racked on the shoulder, extend the knees and hips until you are fully upright.
11. Lower the dumbbell to the starting position and repeat with the other arm.

Common Errors

- Placing the feet either wider or narrower than shoulder width.
- Holding the dumbbells either above or below the knee joint.
- In the start position, placing the shoulders either over or behind the dumbbells instead of slightly in front of them.
- Bending the elbows before the ankles, knees, and hips are fully extended and the shoulders are at the top of the shrug.
- Bringing the dumbbell to the shoulder in an arched movement rather than straight up to the armpits.
- Sitting under the dumbbell by flexing at the knees and bringing them in front of the toes instead of by sitting back at the hips.
- Catching with the elbow pointing toward the floor rather than toward the wall.
- Sitting too deep in the catching action rather than just deep enough to rack the dumbbells on the shoulders.

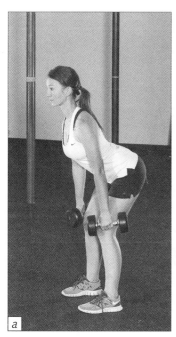
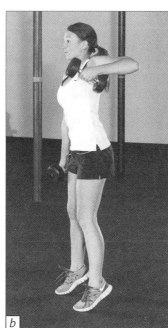
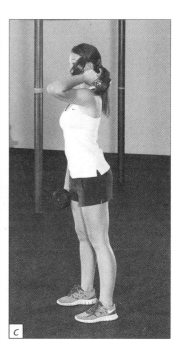

a

b

c

One-Arm Power Clean

Instructions

1. Stand with the feet about shoulder-width apart.
2. With the arms hanging at the sides, hold a dumbbell in the right hand at the side of the right leg.
3. Sit back at the hips, keeping the back arched and the head up, and lower the dumbbell until the handle is positioned at the desired start position height (i.e., with the handle of the dumbbell centered with the knee joint when performing from the hang start position, and from mid-shin when performing the full movement).
4. The shoulders should be slightly in front of the dumbbell. If the shoulders are not in front of the knees, straighten the knees until achieving this position.
5. To begin the lift, push against the ground to extend the hip, knee, and ankle joints.
6. After achieving full extension, aggressively shrug the right shoulder to elevate the dumbbell slightly.
7. Once the shrug is complete, pull the dumbbell along the rib cage to the lower portion of the armpit.
8. From this position, pull the body under the dumbbell by flexing at the hips and aggressively bring the right elbow around to rack the back half of the dumbbell on the right shoulder while catching the dumbbell in a quarter squat position.
9. In this racked position the head should be up and the back arched, the elbow should be high, and the knees should be behind the toes.
10. Once the dumbbell has been racked on the shoulder, extend the knees and hips so that you are fully upright.
11. Lower the dumbbell to the starting position and complete the required number of repetitions.
12. Repeat the exercise on the left arm.

Common Errors

- Placing the feet either wider or narrower than shoulder width.
- Holding the dumbbells either above or below the knee joint.
- In the start position, placing the shoulders either over or behind the dumbbells instead of slightly in front of them.
- Bending the elbow before the ankles, knees, and hips are fully extended and the shoulders are at the top of the shrug.
- Bringing the dumbbell to the shoulder in an arched movement rather than straight up to the armpit.
- Sitting under the dumbbell by flexing at the knees and bringing them in front of the toes instead of by sitting back at the hips.
- Catching with the elbow pointing toward the floor rather than toward the wall.
- Sitting too deep in the catching action rather than just deep enough to rack the dumbbells on the shoulders.

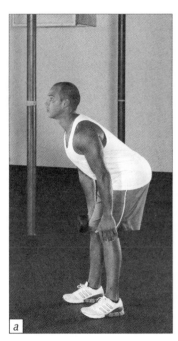 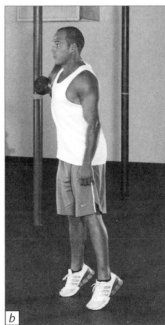 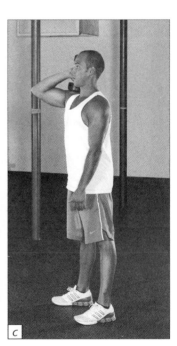

a   b   c

Hang Clean

Instructions

1. Stand with the feet about shoulder-width apart.
2. With the arms hanging at the sides, hold a pair of dumbbells at the sides of the legs.
3. Sit back at the hips, keeping the back arched and the head up, and lower the dumbbells until the handles are positioned at the desired start position height (i.e., with the handle of the dumbbell centered with the knee joint when performing from the hang start position, and from mid-shin when performing the full movement).
4. The shoulders should be slightly in front of the dumbbells.
5. If the shoulders are not in front of the knees, straighten the knees until achieving this position.
6. Initiate the movement by forcefully pushing against the ground to extend the hips, knees, and ankles.
7. After achieving full extension, aggressively shrug the shoulders to elevate the dumbbells slightly.
8. Once the shrug is complete, pull the dumbbells along the rib cage to the lower portion of the armpits.
9. From this position, pull the body under the dumbbells by flexing at the hips and aggressively bringing the elbows around to rack the back half of the dumbbells on the shoulders.
10. Continue to sit back at the hips until you are in a parallel squat position, keeping the heels on the ground.
11. In this racked position the head should be up and the back arched, the elbows should be high, and the knees should be behind the toes.
12. From the full squat position, extend the knees and hips until you are fully upright, keeping the head up and the back arched.

Common Errors

- Placing the feet either wider or narrower than shoulder-width apart.
- Holding the dumbbells either above or below the knee joint.
- In the start position, positioning the shoulders either over or behind the dumbbells rather than slightly in front of the dumbbells.
- Bending the elbows before the ankles, knees, and hips are fully extended and the shoulders are at the top of the shrug.
- Bringing the dumbbells to the shoulders in an arched movement rather than straight up to the armpits.
- Sitting under the dumbbells by flexing at the knees and bringing them in front of the toes instead of by sitting back at the hips.
- Catching with the elbows pointing toward the floor rather than toward the wall.
- Sitting too deep in the catching action rather than just deep enough to rack the dumbbells on the shoulders in a semisquat position.
- Failing to achieve a full parallel squat position.

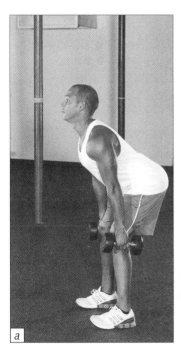
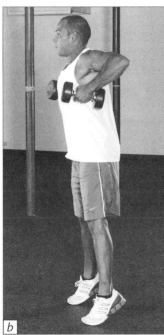
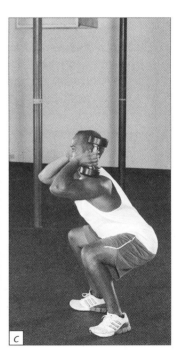

Alternating Hang Clean

Instructions

1. Stand with the feet about shoulder-width apart.
2. With the arms hanging at the sides, hold a pair of dumbbells at the sides of the legs.
3. Sit back at the hips, keeping the back arched and the head up, and lower the dumbbells until the handles are positioned at the desired start position height (i.e., with the handle of the dumbbell centered with the knee joint when performing from the hang start position, and from mid-shin when performing the full movement).
4. The shoulders should be slightly in front of the dumbbells.
5. If the shoulders are not in front of the knees, straighten the knees until achieving this position.
6. Initiate the movement by forcefully pushing against the ground to extend the hips, knees, and ankles.
7. After achieving full extension, aggressively shrug the shoulders to elevate the dumbbells slightly.
8. Once the shrug is complete, pull the dumbbells along the rib cage to the lower portion of the armpits. Alternate this pulling action with each repetition between the right and left arms. Continue to sit back at the hips until you are in a parallel squat position, keeping the heels on the ground.
9. In this racked position the head should be up and the back arched, the elbows should be high, and the knees should be behind the toes.
10. From the full squat position, extend the knees and hips until you are fully upright, keeping the head up and the back arched.
11. Repeat the exercise on the left arm.

Common Errors

- Placing the feet either wider or narrower than shoulder width.
- Holding the dumbbells either above or below the knee joint.
- In the start position, placing the shoulders either over or behind the dumbbells instead of slightly in front of the dumbbells.
- Bending the elbows before the ankles, knees, and hips are fully extended and the shoulders are at the top of the shrug.
- Bringing the dumbbells to the shoulders in an arched movement rather than straight up to the armpits.
- Sitting under the dumbbells by flexing at the knees and bringing them in front of the toes instead of by sitting back at the hips.
- Catching with the elbows pointing toward the floor rather than toward the wall.
- Sitting too deep in the catching action instead of in a semisquat position just deep enough to rack the dumbbells on the shoulders.
- Failing to achieve a full parallel squat position.

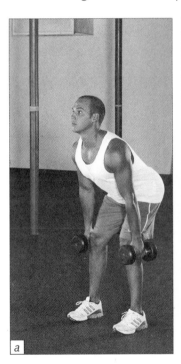

a

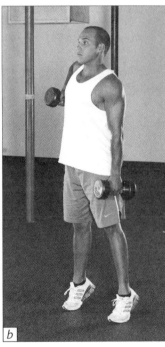

b

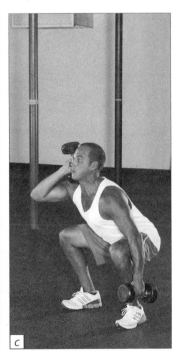

c

One-Arm Hang Clean

Instructions

1. Stand with the feet about shoulder-width apart.
2. Hold a dumbbell in the right hand at the side of the leg.
3. Sit back at the hips, keeping the back arched and the head up, and lower the dumbbell until the handle is positioned at the desired start position height (i.e., with the handle of the dumbbell centered with the knee joint when performing from the hang start position, and from mid-shin when performing the full movement).
4. The shoulders should be slightly in front of the dumbbell.
5. If the shoulders are not in front of the knees, straighten the knees until achieving this position.
6. Initiate the movement by forcefully pushing against the ground to extend the hips, knees, and ankles.
7. After achieving full extension, aggressively shrug the shoulders to elevate the dumbbell slightly.
8. Once the shrug is complete, pull the dumbbell along the rib cage to the lower portion of the armpit.
9. Continue to sit back at the hips until you are in a parallel squat position, and keep the heels on the ground.
10. In this racked position, the head should be up and the back arched, the elbows should be high, and the knees should be behind the toes.
11. From the full squat position, extend the knees and hips until you are fully upright, keeping the head up and the back arched.
12. Repeat the movement with the left arm.

Common Errors

- Placing the feet either wider or narrower than shoulder width.
- Holding the dumbbell either above or below the knee joint.
- In the start position, placing the shoulders either over or behind the dumbbell instead of slightly in front it.
- Bending the elbow before the ankles, knees, and hips are fully extended and the shoulders are at the top of the shrug.
- Bringing the dumbbell to the shoulder in an arched movement rather than straight up to the armpits.
- Sitting under the dumbbell by flexing at the knees and bringing them in front of the toes instead of by sitting back at the hips.
- Catching with the elbow pointing toward the floor rather than toward the wall.
- Sitting too deep in the catching action instead of in a semisquat position just deep enough to rack the dumbbells on the shoulders.
- Failing to achieve a full parallel squat position.

Power Snatch

Instructions

1. Stand with the feet shoulder-width apart.
2. Hold a pair of dumbbells at the sides of the legs.
3. Sit back at the hips, keeping the back arched and the head up, and lower the dumbbells until the handles are positioned at the desired start position height (i.e., with the handle of the dumbbell centered with the knee joint when performing from the hang start position, and from mid-shin when performing the full movement).
4. The shoulders should be slightly in front of the dumbbells.
5. If the shoulders are not in front of the knees, straighten the knees until they are.
6. Initiate the movement by forcefully pushing against the ground to extend the hips, knees, and ankles.
7. After fully extending, aggressively shrug the shoulders to elevate the dumbbells slightly.
8. Once the shrug is complete, pull the dumbbells along the rib cage to the lower portion of the armpits.
9. Continue pulling the dumbbells up in one fluid movement until they are caught directly over the shoulders with the arms fully extended. At the same time, flex the hips to lower the body slightly into a semisquat position when catching the dumbbells.
10. Once the dumbbells have been caught in the fully extended position above the shoulders, extend the knees and hips so you are in a fully upright position and control the dumbbells for a full second before lowering them back to the start position.

Common Errors

- Placing the feet either wider or narrower than shoulder-width apart.
- Holding the dumbbells either above or below the knee joint.
- In the start position, placing the shoulders either over or behind the dumbbells instead of slightly in front of them.
- Bending the elbow before the ankles, knees, and hips are fully extended and the shoulders are at the top of the shrug.
- Bringing the dumbbells overhead in an arched movement rather than straight up past the hips, shoulder, and ears.
- Sitting under the dumbbells by flexing at the knees and bringing them in front of the toes instead of by sitting back at the hips.
- Failing to control the dumbbells and bring them to a complete stop before lowering them to the start position.

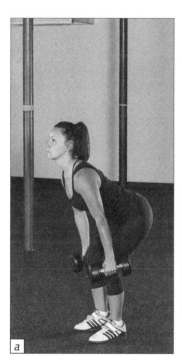
a

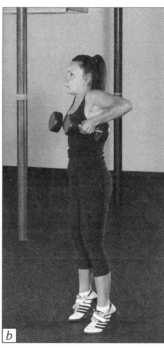
b

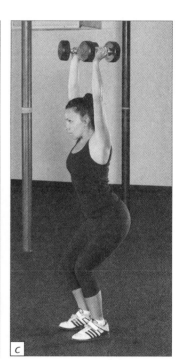
c

Alternating Power Snatch

Instructions

1. Stand with the feet shoulder-width apart.
2. Hold a pair of dumbbells at the sides of the legs.
3. Sit back at the hips, keeping the back arched and the head up, and lower the dumbbells until the handles are positioned at the desired start position height (i.e., with the handle of the dumbbell centered with the knee joint when performing from the hang start position, and from mid-shin when performing the full movement).
4. The shoulders should be slightly in front of the dumbbells.
5. If the shoulders are not in front of the knees, straighten the knees until they are.
6. Initiate the movement by forcefully pushing against the ground to extend the hips, knees, and ankles.
7. After fully extending, aggressively shrug the shoulders to elevate the dumbbells slightly.
8. Once the shrug is complete pull the dumbbell in the right hand along the rib cage to the lower portion of the armpit.
9. Continue pulling the dumbbell up in one fluid movement until it is caught directly over the right shoulder with the right arm fully extended. At the same time, flex the hips to lower the body slightly into a semisquat position when catching the dumbbell.
10. Once the dumbbell has been caught in the fully extended position above the left shoulder, extend the knees and hips so you are fully upright. Control the dumbbell for a full second before lowering it to the start position.
11. Repeat the movement with the left arm.

Common Errors

- Placing the feet either wider or narrower than shoulder-width apart.
- Holding the dumbbells either above or below the knee joint.
- In the start position, placing the shoulders either over or behind the dumbbells instead of slightly in front of them.
- Bending the elbow before the ankles, knees, and hips are fully extended and the shoulders are at the top of the shrug.
- Bringing the dumbbell overhead in an arched movement rather than straight up past the hips, shoulder, and ears.
- Sitting under the dumbbell by flexing at the knees and bringing them front of the toes instead of by sitting back at the hips.
- Failing to control the dumbbell and bring it to a complete stop before lowering it to the start position.

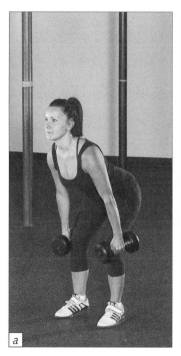
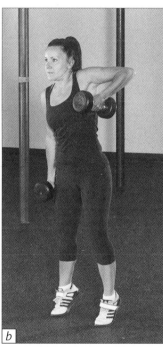
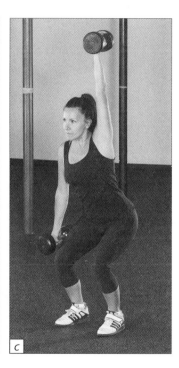

a

b

c

One-Arm Power Snatch

Instructions

1. Stand with the feet shoulder-width apart.
2. Hold a dumbbell in the right hand at the side of the right leg.
3. Sit back at the hips, keeping the back arched and the head up, and lower the dumbbell until the handle is positioned at the desired start position height (i.e., with the handle of the dumbbell centered with the knee joint when performing from the hang start position, and from mid-shin when performing the full movement).
4. The shoulders should be slightly in front of the dumbbell.
5. If the shoulders are not in front of the knees, straighten the knees until they are.
6. Initiate the movement by forcefully pushing against the ground to extend the hips, knees, and ankles.
7. After fully extending, aggressively shrug the right shoulder to elevate the dumbbell slightly.
8. Once the shrug is complete, pull the dumbbell in the right hand along the rib cage to the lower portion of the armpit.
9. Continue pulling the dumbbell up in one fluid movement until it is caught directly over the right shoulder with the right arm fully extended. At the same time flex the hips to lower the body slightly into a semisquat position upon catching the dumbbell.
10. Once the dumbbell has been caught in the fully extended position above the right shoulder, extend the knees and hips so you are fully upright. Control the dumbbell for a full second before lowering it to the start position.
11. Repeat the movement with the left arm.

Common Errors

- Placing the feet either wider or narrower than shoulder-width apart.
- Holding the dumbbell either above or below the knee joint.
- In the start position, placing the shoulders either over or behind the dumbbell instead of slightly in front of it.
- Bending the elbow before the ankles, knees, and hips are fully extended and the shoulders are at the top of the shrug.
- Bringing the dumbbell overhead in an arched movement rather than straight up past the hips, shoulder, and ears.
- Sitting under the dumbbell by flexing at the knees and bringing them in front of the toes instead of by sitting back at the hips.
- Failing to control the dumbbell and bring it to a complete stop before lowering it back to the start position.

Split Alternating-Feet Snatch

Instructions

1. Stand with the feet shoulder-width apart.
2. Hold a pair of dumbbells at the sides of the legs.
3. Sit back at the hips, keeping the back arched and the head up, and lower the dumbbells until the handles are positioned at the desired start position height (i.e., with the handle of the dumbbell centered with the knee joint when performing from the hang start position, and from mid-shin when performing the full movement).
4. The shoulders should be slightly in front of the dumbbells.
5. If the shoulders are not in front of the knees, straighten the knees until they are.
6. Initiate the movement by forcefully pushing against the ground to extend the hips, knees, and ankles.
7. After fully extending, aggressively shrug the shoulders to elevate the dumbbells slightly.
8. Once the shrug is complete, pull the dumbbells along the rib cage to the lower portion of the armpits.
9. Continue pulling the dumbbells up in one fluid movement until they are caught directly over the shoulders with the arms fully extended. At the same time, split the legs in a high lunge position, with the left leg moving forward and the right leg moving back.
10. Once the dumbbells have been caught in the fully extended position above the shoulders, recover the feet to the start position, stepping up with the left foot and back with the right foot to bring the feet together. Pause briefly in this position.
11. Once the feet have been brought together, lower the dumbbells to the start position and repeat, alternating the feet in the split position each repetition.

Common Errors

- Placing the feet either wider or narrower than shoulder-width apart.
- Holding the dumbbells either above or below the knee joint.
- In the start position, placing the shoulders either over or behind the dumbbells instead of slightly in front of them.
- Bending the elbow before the ankles, knees, and hips are fully extended and the shoulders are at the top of the shrug.
- Bringing the dumbbells overhead in an arched movement rather than straight up past the hips, shoulder, and ears.
- Failing to move the front foot far enough forward in the split to lower the body under the dumbbells.
- Failing to control the dumbbells and bring them to a complete stop before lowering them to the start position.
- Lowering the dumbbells before fully recovering the feet to the start position.

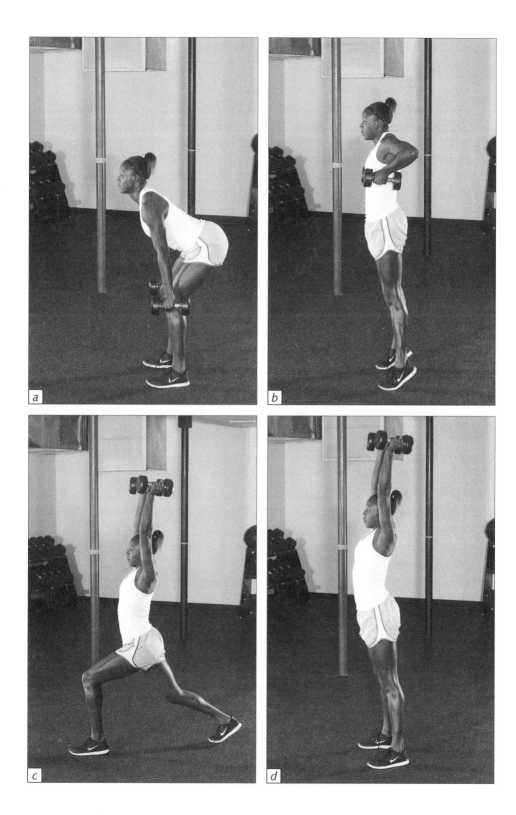

Split Alternating-Feet Alternating-Arm Snatch

Instructions

1. Stand with the feet shoulder-width apart.
2. Hold a pair of dumbbells at the sides of the legs.
3. Sit back at the hips, keeping the back arched and the head up, and lower the dumbbells until the handles are positioned at the desired start position height (i.e., with the handle of the dumbbell centered with the knee joint when performing from the hang start position, and from mid-shin when performing the full movement).
4. The shoulders should be slightly in front of the dumbbells.
5. If the shoulders are not in front of the knees, straighten the knees until they are.
6. Initiate the movement by forcefully pushing against the ground to extend the hips, knees, and ankles.
7. After fully extending, aggressively shrug the shoulders to elevate the dumbbells slightly.
8. Once the shrug is complete, pull the dumbbell in the right hand along the rib cage to the lower portion of the armpit.
9. Continue pulling the dumbbell up in one fluid movement until it is caught directly over the right shoulder with the right arm fully extended. At the same time, split the legs in a high lunge position, with the left leg moving forward and the right leg moving back.
10. Once the dumbbells have been caught in the fully extended position over the shoulder, recover the feet to the start position, stepping up with the right foot and stepping back with the left foot to bring the feet together. Pause briefly in this position.
11. Once the feet have been brought together, lower the dumbbell to the start position and repeat, alternating arms and the feet in the split position each repetition.

Common Errors

- Placing the feet either wider or narrower than shoulder-width apart.
- Holding the dumbbells either above or below the knee joint.
- In the start position, positioning the shoulders either over or behind the dumbbells instead of slightly in front of them.
- Bending the elbow before the ankles, knees, and hips are fully extended and the shoulders are at the top of the shrug.
- Bringing the dumbbell overhead in an arched movement rather than straight up past the hips, shoulder, and ears.
- Failing to move the front foot far enough forward in the split to lower the body under the dumbbells.
- Failing to control the dumbbell and bring it to a complete stop before lowering it back to the start position.
- Lowering the dumbbell before fully recovering the feet to the start position.

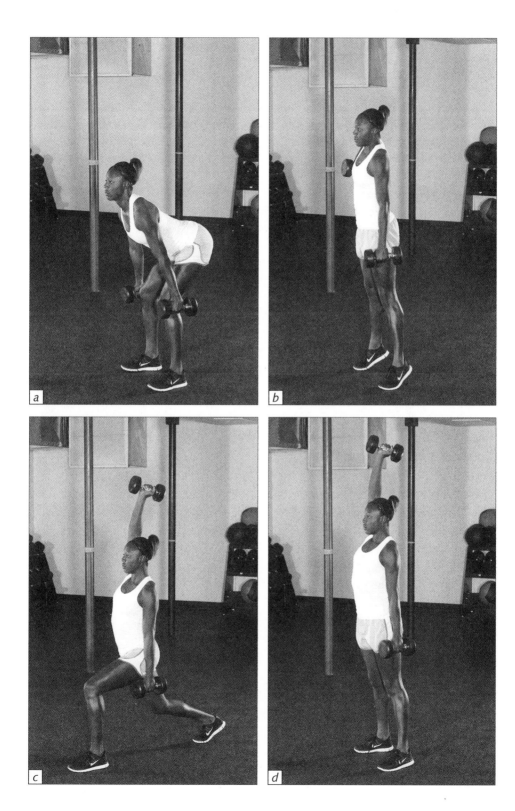

One-Arm Split Alternating-Feet Snatch

Instructions

1. Stand with the feet shoulder-width apart.
2. Hold a dumbbell in the left hand with the arm hanging down along the side of the leg.
3. Sit back at the hips, keeping the back arched and the head up, and lower the dumbbell until the handle is at the desired start position height (i.e., with the handle of the dumbbell centered with the knee joint when performing from the hang start position, and from mid-shin when performing the full movement).
4. The shoulders should be slightly in front of the dumbbell.
5. If the shoulders are not in front of the knees, straighten the knees until they are.
6. Initiate the movement by forcefully pushing against the ground to extend the hips, knees, and ankles.
7. After fully extending, aggressively shrug the shoulder to raise the dumbbell slightly.
8. Once the shrug is complete, pull the dumbbell in the right hand along the rib cage to the lower portion of the armpit.
9. Continue pulling the dumbbell up in one fluid movement until it is caught directly over the left shoulder with the arm fully extended. At the same time, split the legs in a high lunge position, with the left leg moving forward and the right leg moving back.
10. Once the dumbbell has been caught in the fully extended position above the shoulder, recover the feet to the start position, stepping up with the left foot and stepping back with the right foot to bring the feet together. Pause briefly in this position.
11. Once the feet are together, lower the dumbbell to the start position and repeat, alternating the split position each repetition.

Common Errors

- Placing the feet either wider or narrower than shoulder-width apart.
- Holding the dumbbell either above or below the knee joint.
- In the start position, positioning the shoulders either over or behind the dumbbell instead of slightly in front of it.
- Bending the elbow before the ankles, knees, and hips are fully extended and the shoulders are at the top of the shrug.
- Bringing the dumbbell overhead in an arched movement rather than straight up past the hips, shoulder, and ears.
- Failing to move the front foot far enough forward in the split to lower the body under the dumbbells.
- Failing to control the dumbbell and bring it to a complete stop before lowering it to the start position.
- Lowering the dumbbell before fully recovering the feet to the start position.

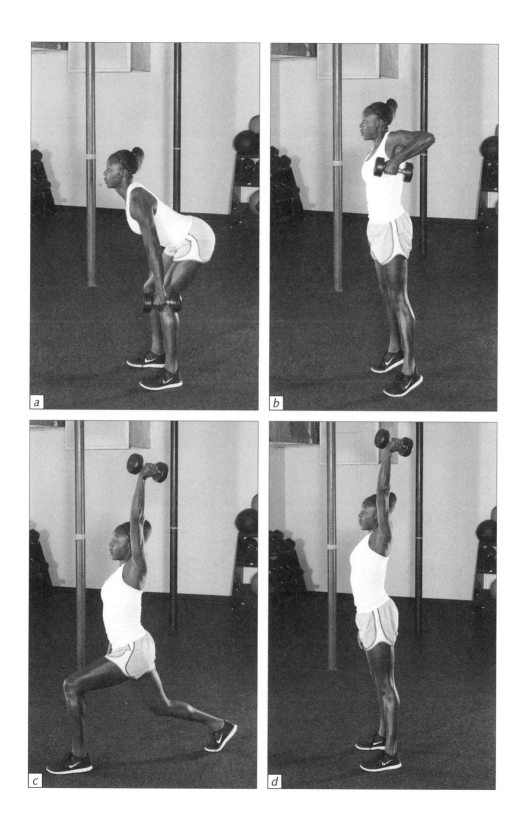

PART III

PROGRAMMING

Once you understand the benefits of dumbbell training and are familiar with the exercises that can be performed using this mode of training, you can now initiate the process of designing a resistance training program meant to achieve your specific goals. The final five chapters take a look at programming, first for the physiological adaptations of increased muscle size and power, and then for specific types of sports. These are grouped into power, speed, and balance sports. Because it would be impossible to discuss every sport, the workouts for each of the three categories are examples for sports that share similar characteristics. For example, the power sport chapter includes training programs for throwers in track and field events and for basketball and volleyball players. Although each of these activities requires different physiological attributes, they all require a high level of muscular power for optimal performance.

By reviewing the information on training for power and then seeing how that information has been applied in the sample workouts, you should be able to design a training program for other sports that require power, such as football or pole vault. The same process can be applied to speed or balance sports. Begin by writing your program based on the requirements of the sport using the information provided, implement the program, and then revise it based on the results you achieve. Revising your workouts is a never-ending process of working towards developing the best program possible. As you continue to refine your program, make sure you make programming decisions based on your current training status and not where you want to be. Avoid the mistake of looking ahead to your future goals and making programming decisions based on what you hope to accomplish. This approach can lead to designing workouts you are not ready for and to potential injury and frustration.

CHAPTER 8

Training for Increased Muscle Size

Training for increases in muscle size (hypertrophy) is a common goal among people who lift weights, either for aesthetic reasons or as a way to improve athletic performance. When your goal is hypertrophy, it is a good idea to look at the experiences of lifters in the gym and also to see what science has to say about building muscle mass. This combination of real-world observation backed up with scientific research is a good approach to solving any problem and certainly provides a sound foundation for program design.

If you look at the training programs used by most bodybuilders, who are judged primarily by the amount of muscle mass they have developed, you will find recurring practices. Most bodybuilders perform exercise repetitions in a range of 8 to 12. Yes, some may be a little higher and some a little lower, but in general this is the range. Most bodybuilders perform multiple sets, typically four to six sets per exercise. These four to six sets of 8 to 12 repetitions are generally separated by rests of 60 to 90 seconds. This protocol has been used successfully for years to increase muscle mass.

This approach is supported by science. Research shows that a combination of short rests and high repetitions results in elevated levels of testosterone, human growth hormone, and insulin-like growth hormone when comparing preexercise levels to postexercise. Each of these hormones is important in bringing about hypertrophy.

In addition to performing 8 to 12 repetitions over four to six sets, and using rest times of 60 to 90 seconds, training must be sufficiently intense to cause adaptation. Rather than using a percentage system, I designate the desired intensity based on the number of repetitions to be performed (i.e., repetition maximum). In the case of developing hypertrophy, where it is advantageous to keep the training volume high, we require a training resistance as high as possible while allowing completion of the full number of repetitions performed using good technique. Because of the short rest times between sets, you may need to slightly reduce the resistance as you progress through the sets to be able to complete the full number of repetitions in each set.

An additional suggestion when training for hypertrophy is to emphasize multijoint exercises (e.g., squats) over single-joint exercises (e.g., leg extensions). This produces two primary advantages. First, the more muscle mass you recruit, the more muscle mass you stimulate to increase in size. Squats primarily recruit the muscles of the quadriceps, hamstrings, glutes, and the lower back. In contrast, leg extensions recruit the quads only. Second, the greater the amount of muscle mass recruited, the greater the hormonal response will be. A greater hormonal response increases the opportunity for optimal increases in muscle mass.

Because the Olympic lifts are performed explosively, typically with low repetitions and extended rest times to emphasize speed of movement and technique, they are not emphasized when the goal of training is hypertrophy. However, these movements can be manipulated to provide a greater hypertrophic response by performing compound exercises. So, for example, you can perform dumbbell power cleans to a squat to a power jerk. In this example, the lifter first performs a dumbbell power clean. At the completion of the power clean, the lifter racks the dumbbells on the shoulders and performs a front squat taken to parallel or lower. At the top of the front squat, the lifter stops and then performs a power jerk. Putting these movements together significantly increases the amount of muscle mass recruited and thus enhances the potential hypertrophic response. This is just one example of total-body exercises that can be combined.

In summary, when training for hypertrophy, perform four to six sets of 8 to 12 repetitions with 60 to 90 seconds of recovery between sets and exercises. Choose a resistance that is at or just short of repetition maximum and emphasize multiple-joint exercises.

SAMPLE WORKOUT SCHEDULES

Now let's look at sample workouts. The first workout emphasizes hypertrophy only, so the training variables have been manipulated to achieve that goal. The second sample workout emphasizes hypertrophy as its primary goal, but has a second goal of increasing strength. This workout includes two sets of training variables. One set of training variables is manipulated to bring about increases in hypertrophy, and the second set is manipulated to increase in strength.

Hypertrophy Cycle

Monday

Length 5 weeks

Goal Increase muscle size.

Intensity Complete the full number of required repetitions on each set.

Pace Perform total-body lifts explosively. On all other exercises lift as explosively as possible and lower in 3 seconds.

Rest Take 1:30 between total-body exercise sets and 1:00 between all other sets and exercises.

Set and Reps

Week	Hypertrophy
1	TB = 4 × 6 CL = 4 × 8 AL = 3 × 10
2	TB = 4 × 4 CL = 4 × 10 AL = 3 × 10
3	TB = 4 × 6 CL = 4 × 8 AL = 3 × 10
4	TB = 4 × 5 CL = 4 × 12 AL = 3 × 10
5	TB = 4 × 3 CL = 4 × 6 AL = 3 × 10

	Week 1	Week 2	Week 3	Week 4	Week 5
TOTAL BODY					
Power jerk TB	4 × 6	4 × 4	4 × 6	4 × 4	4 × 6
Weight lifted					
LOWER BODY					
Front squat CL	4 × 8	4 × 10	4 × 8	4 × 12	4 × 6
Weight lifted					
SLDL CL	4 × 8	4 × 10	4 × 8	4 × 12	4 × 6
Weight lifted					
TRUNK					
Crunch	3 × 20	3 × 20	3 × 20	3 × 20	3 × 20
Weight lifted					
Back extension	3 × 12	3 × 12	3 × 12	3 × 12	3 × 12
Weight lifted					
UPPER BACK					
Row CL	4 × 8	4 × 10	4 × 8	4 × 10	4 × 6
Weight lifted					
Bent lateral raise AL	3 × 10	3 × 10	3 × 10	3 × 10	3 × 10
Weight lifted					

Note: The following abbreviations are used in the workout tables. TB = total body, one of the Olympic-style lifts or related training exercise; CL = core lift, a multijoint exercise such as a squat; AL = auxiliary lift, a single-joint exercise such as a biceps curl; SLDL = straight-leg deadlift; alt = the exercise is performed alternating legs or alternating arms.

(continued)

Hypertrophy Cycle *(continued)*

Wednesday

Length   5 weeks

Goal   Increase muscle size.

Intensity   Complete the full number of required repetitions on each set.

Pace   Perform total-body lifts explosively. In all other exercises lift as explosively as possible and lower in 3 seconds.

Rest   Take 1:30 between total-body exercise sets and 1:00 between all other sets and exercises.

Sets and Reps

Week	Hypertrophy
1	TB = 4 × 6 CL = 4 × 8 AL = 3 × 10
2	TB = 4 × 4 CL = 4 × 10 AL = 3 × 10
3	TB = 4 × 6 CL = 4 × 8 AL = 3 × 10
4	TB = 4 × 5 CL = 4 × 12 AL = 3 × 10
5	TB = 4 × 3 CL = 4 × 6 AL = 3 × 10

	Week 1	Week 2	Week 3	Week 4	Week 5
TOTAL BODY					
Hang power clean TB	4 × 6	4 × 4	4 × 6	4 × 4	4 × 6
Weight lifted					
LOWER BODY					
Squat CL	4 × 8	4 × 10	4 × 8	4 × 12	4 × 6
Weight lifted					
Lateral squat CL	4 × 8	4 × 10	4 × 8	4 × 12	4 × 6
Weight lifted					
TRUNK					
Twist crunch	3 × 20	3 × 20	3 × 20	3 × 20	3 × 20
Weight lifted					
Alt toe touch	3 × 20	3 × 20	3 × 20	3 × 20	3 × 20
Weight lifted					
UPPER BODY					
Bench press CL	4 × 8	4 × 10	4 × 8	4 × 12	4 × 6
Weight lifted					
Fly AL	3 × 10	3 × 10	3 × 10	3 × 10	3 × 10
Weight lifted					

Friday

Length 5 weeks

Goal Increase muscle size.

Intensity Complete the full number of required repetitions on each set.

Pace Perform total-body lifts explosively. In all other exercises lift as explosively as possible and lower in 3 seconds.

Rest Take 1:30 between total-body exercise sets and 1:00 between all other sets and exercises.

Sets and Reps

Week	Hypertrophy
1	TB = 4 × 6 CL = 4 × 8 AL = 3 × 10
2	TB = 4 × 4 CL = 4 × 10 AL = 3 × 10
3	TB = 4 × 6 CL = 4 × 8 AL = 3 × 10
4	TB = 4 × 5 CL = 4 × 12 AL = 3 × 10
5	TB = 4 × 3 CL = 4 × 6 AL = 3 × 10

	Week 1	Week 2	Week 3	Week 4	Week 5
TOTAL BODY					
Power snatch TB	4 × 6	4 × 4	4 × 6	4 × 5	4 × 3
Weight lifted					
TRUNK					
V-up	3 × 20	3 × 20	3 × 20	3 × 20	3 × 20
Weight lifted					
Twist back extension	3 × 12	3 × 12	3 × 12	3 × 12	3 × 12
Weight lifted					
CHEST					
Incline press CL	4 × 8	4 × 10	4 × 8	4 × 12	4 × 6
Weight lifted					
Incline fly AL	3 × 10	3 × 10	3 × 10	3 × 10	3 × 10
Weight lifted					
SHOULDERS					
Shoulder press CL	4 × 8	4 × 10	4 × 8	4 × 12	4 × 6
Weight lifted					
Lateral raise AL	3 × 10	3 × 10	3 × 10	3 × 10	3 × 10
Weight lifted					

Hypertrophy and Strength Cycle

Monday (Hypertrophy)

Length   5 weeks

Goals   To increase muscle size and strength.

Intensity   Hypertrophy: Complete the full number of required repetitions on each set. Strength: Complete the full number of required repetitions on the first set only.

Pace   Perform total-body lifts explosively. Hypertrophy: In all other exercises, lift as explosively as possible and lower in 3 seconds. Strength: Lower in 2 seconds.

Rest   Hypertrophy: Take 1:30 between total-body exercise sets and 1:00 between all other sets and exercises. Strength: Take 2:00 between all sets and exercises.

Sets and Reps

Week	Hypertrophy	Strength
1	TB = 4 × 6 CL = 4 × 8 AL = 3 × 10	TB = 4 × 3 CL = 4 × 5 AL = 3 × 8
2	TB = 4 × 4 CL = 4 × 10 AL = 3 × 10	TB = 4 × 5 CL = 4 × 7 AL = 3 × 8
3	TB = 4 × 6 CL = 4 × 8 AL = 3 × 10	TB = 4 × 3 CL = 4 × 4 AL = 3 × 8
4	TB = 4 × 5 CL = 4 × 12 AL = 3 × 10	TB = 4 × 5 CL = 4 × 6 AL = 3 × 8
5	TB = 4 × 3 CL = 4 × 6 AL = 3 × 10	TB = 4 × 2 CL = 4 × 4 AL = 3 × 8

	Week 1	Week 2	Week 3	Week 4	Week 5
TOTAL BODY					
Hang power clean TB	4 × 6	4 × 4	4 × 6	4 × 4	4 × 6
Weight lifted					
LOWER BODY					
Squat CL	4 × 8	4 × 10	4 × 8	4 × 10	4 × 8
Weight lifted					
SLDL CL	4 × 8	4 × 10	4 × 8	4 × 10	4 × 8
Weight lifted					
TRUNK					
Alt V-up	3 × 20	3 × 30	3 × 20	3 × 20	3 × 20
Weight lifted					
Back extension	3 × 12	3 × 12	3 × 12	3 × 12	3 × 12
Weight lifted					
UPPER BACK					
Row	4 × 8	4 × 10	4 × 8	4 × 10	4 × 8
Weight lifted					
Bent lateral raise AL	3 × 10	3 × 10	3 × 10	3 × 10	3 × 10
Weight lifted					

Wednesday (Strength)

Length 5 weeks

Goals Increase muscle size and strength.

Intensity Hypertrophy: Complete the full number of required repetitions on each set. Strength: Complete the full number of required repetitions on the first set only.

Pace Perform total-body lifts explosively. Hypertrophy: In all other exercises lift as explosively as possible and lower in 3 seconds Strength: Lower in 2 seconds.

Rest Hypertrophy: Take 1:30 between total-body exercise sets and 1:00 between all other sets and exercises. Strength: Take 2:00 between all sets and exercises.

Sets and Reps

Week	Hypertrophy	Strength
1	TB = 4 × 6 CL = 4 × 8	TB = 4 × 3 CL = 4 × 5
2	TB = 4 × 4 CL = 4 × 10	TB = 4 × 5 CL = 4 × 7
3	TB = 4 × 6 CL = 4 × 8	TB = 4 × 3 CL = 4 × 4
4	TB = 4 × 5 CL = 4 × 12	TB = 4 × 5 CL = 4 × 6
5	TB = 4 × 3 CL = 4 × 6	TB = 4 × 2 CL = 4 × 4

	Week 1	Week 2	Week 3	Week 4	Week 5
TOTAL BODY					
Push press TB	4 × 3	4 × 5	4 × 3	4 × 5	4 × 3
Weight lifted					
LOWER BODY					
Squat CL	4 × 5	4 × 7	4 × 5	4 × 7	4 × 5
Weight lifted					
Lateral squat CL	4 × 5	4 × 7	4 × 5	4 × 7	4 × 5
Weight lifted					
TRUNK					
Crunch	3 × 15	3 × 15	3 × 15	3 × 15	3 × 15
Weight lifted					
Twisting back extension	3 × 10	3 × 10	3 × 10	3 × 10	3 × 10
Weight lifted					
UPPER BODY					
Incline press CL	4 × 5	4 ×7	4 × 5	4 × 7	4 × 5
Weight lifted					
Shoulder press CL	4 × 5	4 × 7	4 × 5	4 × 7	4 × 5
Weight lifted					

(continued)

Hypertrophy and Strength Cycle *(continued)*

Friday (Hypertrophy)

Length   5 weeks

Goals   Increase muscle size and strength.

Intensity   Hypertrophy: Complete the full number of required repetitions on each set. Strength: Complete the full number of required repetitions on the first set only.

Pace   Perform total-body lifts explosively. Hypertrophy: In all other exercises lift as explosively as possible and lower in 3 seconds. Strength: Lower in 2 seconds.

Rest   Hypertrophy: Take 1:30 between total-body exercise sets and 1:00 between all other sets and exercises. Strength: Take 2:00 between all sets and exercises.

Sets and Reps

Week	Hypertrophy	Strength
1	TB = 4 × 6 CL = 4 × 8	TB = 4 × 3 CL = 4 × 5
2	TB = 4 × 4 CL = 4 × 10	TB = 4 × 5 CL = 4 × 7
3	TB = 4 × 6 CL = 4 × 8	TB = 4 × 3 CL = 4 × 4
4	TB = 4 × 5 CL = 4 × 12	TB = 4 × 5 CL = 4 × 6
5	TB = 4 × 3 CL = 4 × 6	TB = 4 × 2 CL = 4 × 4

	Week 1	Week 2	Week 3	Week 4	Week 5
TOTAL BODY					
Power snatch TB	4 × 6	4 × 4	4 × 6	4 × 4	4 × 6
Weight lifted					
UPPER BODY					
Bench press CL	4 × 8	4 × 10	4 × 8	4 × 10	4 × 8
Weight lifted					
Fly CL	4 × 8	4 × 10	4 × 8	4 × 10	4 × 8
Weight lifted					
TRUNK					
Toe touch	3 × 20	3 × 30	3 × 20	3 × 20	3 × 20
Weight lifted					
Twisting crunch	3 × 20	3 × 30	3 × 20	3 × 20	3 × 20
Weight lifted					
UPPER BACK					
Row	4 × 8	4 × 10	4 × 8	4 × 10	4 × 8
Weight lifted					
Upright row CL	4 × 8	4 × 10	4 × 8	4 × 10	4 × 8
Weight lifted					

CHAPTER 9

Training for Increased Power

Before we can talk about training for increased power, we have to establish a working definition of power. Power can be calculated in two ways: as work divided by time or as force multiplied by velocity and measured in watts. In most sports and for most athletes, the ability to generate power is a key to successful performance. Think of a basketball player jumping high over the rim to dunk a basketball player, a sprinter exploding out of the starting blocks, or a defensive lineman fighting through a block to sack the quarterback. These are all examples of being able to exert a high amount of force in a short time period that occur in athletics. However, the need to be able to perform powerful movements is not limited to sports. For example, the ability to recover your balance after slipping requires the ability to move powerfully. Falls in the elderly population are more common because they often times lack the power to regain their balance after tripping or slipping.

Training for power should be based on the specific needs of the sport or activity you are preparing for. For example, both a volleyball player and a wrestler need to be powerful. However, the physical needs of these two sports are different. The only resistance a volleyball player encounters during competition is his or her own body weight and the weight of the ball. In contrast, a wrestler has to overcome not only his own body weight but also, because wrestling is a contact sport, the body weight and force generation of the opponent. Therefore, the volleyball player can focus on relatively high-speed training with light weight during training cycles leading up to the competitive phase. The wrestler, on the other hand, will emphasize force generation and high-velocity training to meet the power requirements of the sport.

Before designing a training program to increase power, evaluate the requirements of the sport or activity. The two examples provided, volleyball and wrestling, might be considered to be on opposite ends of the continuum, with volleyball requiring less force generation and a greater velocity component and wrestling a greater force generation requirement and less velocity. This is further complicated by the fact that you must consider the requirements of the positions within a sport. A wrestler in a light weight class will focus on higher-velocity training than a heavyweight will. And wrestlers in the heavier weight classes will emphasize force generation capability more than lightweights will. So there are not only sport-to-sport differences but also differences within a sport.

To train for power, the workout should consist of one to six repetitions and extended rest times of two to three minutes or longer between sets and exercises. While the reps are fewer and the rest is longer than when training for increased muscle size, the primary difference in programs for developing power is the training load. To continue the example of the volleyball player and wrestler, the volleyball player might use training loads between 30 and 60 percent of one-repetition maximum (1RM) to emphasize the training velocity, and the heavyweight wrestler might use training loads of 80 to 100 percent of 1RM training to emphasize force generation while still attempting to move the resistance as quickly as possible. In terms of exercise selection, the exercises should mimic the movements of the sport or activity as closely as possible. In most cases this means selecting exercises that use barbells or dumbbells to perform multijoint exercises in a standing position.

Another training component you can use during a power cycle is timed exercises. In a timed exercise the athlete must complete the repetitions in a certain amount of time. This component changes the focus from how much an athlete can lift to how quickly he or she can lift it. When performing a timed exercise, the protocol is to go as heavy as possible while still completing the required number of repetitions in good form. The athlete stops the set when the time is up, not when the required repetitions have been completed. The athlete increases the weight if he or she completes more than the required repetitions. If fewer than the required number of repetitions are completed, the athlete is instructed to increase the movement speed. If the athlete is still unsuccessful at completing the full number of required repetitions after attempting to increase the movement speed, the resistance should be decreased. When looking at the workouts including the timed lifts you will see, for example, the following information: TL = 3 x 5 @ 9 sec (1.8). The TL indicates that this is a timed lift. The lifter will be performing three sets of five repetitions. On each of the three sets of five repetitions the lifter will have nine seconds to complete the five repetitions. The 1.8 in parenthesis indicates the lifter has 1.8 seconds to complete each of the five repetitions to be able to finish five repetitions in nine seconds (e.g., 5 x 1.8 = 9).

SAMPLE WORKOUT SCHEDULES

With the protocol for training for power established, let's look at sample workouts emphasizing dumbbells when the training goal is power development. The first workout focuses on power only. The training variables have been adjusted based on the guidelines just described for increasing muscular power. The second sample workout focuses primarily on muscular power but has a secondary goal of increasing muscular endurance. In the second workout are two sets of training variables. The first set of training variables are manipulated to increase muscular power. The second set of variables is manipulated to increase muscular endurance.

Power Cycle

Monday

Length   5 weeks

Goal   Increase muscular power.

Intensity   On total-body lifts complete the full number of required repetitions on the first set only. On timed exercises complete the full number of required repetitions in the specified time.

Pace   Perform total-body lifts explosively. In all other exercises lift the weight as explosively as possible to complete the required number of repetitions in the specified time.

Rest   Take 2:30 between total-body sets and exercises and 2:00 between all other sets and exercises.

Sets and Reps

Week	Power
1	TB = 4 × 2 TL = 3 × 5 @ 9 sec
2	TB = 4 × 3 TL = 3 × 3 @ 5 sec
3	TB = 4 × 2 TL = 3 × 5 @ 9 sec
4	TB = 4 × 3 TL = 3 × 3 @ 5 sec
5	TB = 4 × 2 TL = 3 × 5 @ 9 sec

	Week 1	Week 2	Week 3	Week 4	Week 5
PLYOMETRIC					
Box jump	3 × 6	3 × 6	3 × 6	3 × 6	3 × 6
Reps completed					
TOTAL BODY					
Power jerk TB	4 × 2	4 × 3	4 × 2	4 × 3	4 × 2
Weight lifted					
LOWER BODY					
Squat TL	3 × 5 @ 9 sec	3 × 3 @ 5 sec	3 × 5 @ 9 sec	3 × 3 @ 5 sec	3 × 5 @ 9 sec
Weight lifted					
Side lunge TL	3 × 5 @ 9 sec	3 × 3 @ 5 sec	3 × 5 @ 9 sec	3 × 3 @ 5 sec	3 × 5 @ 9 sec
Weight lifted					
TRUNK					
Decline press crunch	3 × 12	3 × 12	3 × 12	3 × 12	3 × 12
Weight lifted					
SLDL TL	3 × 5 @ 9 sec	3 × 3 @ 5 sec	3 × 5 @ 9 sec	3 × 3 @ 5 sec	3 × 5 @ 9 sec
Weight lifted					
UPPER BACK					
Row TL	3 × 5 @ 9 sec	3 × 3 @ 5 sec	3 × 5 @ 9 sec	3 × 3 @ 5 sec	3 × 5 @ 9 sec
Weight lifted					

Note: The following abbreviations are used in the workout tables. TB = total body, one of the Olympic-style lifts or related training exercise; CL = core lift, a multijoint exercise such as a squat; TL = timed lift, the athlete completes the required reps in a specified time; MB = medicine ball, the exercise is performed with a medicine ball (medicine balls are often used in training programs when the goal of training is to develop power, because medicine balls are designed to be thrown explosively); SLDL = straight-leg deadlift; alt = the exercise is performed alternating legs or alternating arms.

Wednesday

Length 5 weeks

Goal Increase muscular power.

Intensity On total-body lifts complete the full number of required repetitions on the first set only. On timed exercises complete the full number of required repetitions in the specified time.

Pace Perform total-body lifts explosively. In all other exercises lift the weight as explosively as possible to complete the required number of repetitions in the specified time.

Rest Take 2:30 between total-body sets and exercises and 2:00 between all other sets and exercises.

Sets and Reps

Week	Power
1	TB = 4 × 2 TL = 3 × 5 @ 9 sec
2	TB = 4 × 3 TL = 3 × 3 @ 5 sec
3	TB = 4 × 2 TL = 3 × 5 @ 9 sec
4	TB = 4 × 3 TL = 3 × 3 @ 5 sec
5	TB = 4 × 2 TL = 3 × 5 @ 9 sec

	Week 1	Week 2	Week 3	Week 4	Week 5
PLYOMETRIC					
MB lying chest pass	3 × 6	3 × 6	3 × 6	3 × 6	3 × 6
Reps completed					
TOTAL BODY					
Hang clean TB	4 × 2	4 × 3	4 × 2	4 × 3	4 × 2
Weight lifted					
UPPER BODY					
Bench press TL	3 × 5 @ 9 sec	3 × 3 @ 5 sec	3 × 5 @ 9 sec	3 × 3 @ 5 sec	3 × 5 @ 9 sec
Weight lifted					
TRUNK					
Alt V-up	3 × 12	3 × 12	3 × 12	3 × 12	3 × 12
Weight lifted					
SHOULDERS					
Shoulder press TL	3 × 5 @ 9 sec	3 × 3 @ 5 sec	3 × 5 @ 9 sec	3 × 3 @ 5 sec	3 × 5 @ 9 sec
Weight lifted					
Upright row TL	3 × 5 @ 9 sec	3 × 3 @ 5 sec	3 × 5 @ 9 sec	3 × 3 @ 5 sec	3 × 5 @ 9 sec
Weight lifted					

(continued)

Power Cycle *(continued)*

Friday

Length   5 weeks

Goal   Increase muscular power.

Intensity   On total-body lifts complete the full number of required repetitions on the first set only. On timed exercises complete the full number of required repetitions in the specified time.

Pace   Perform total-body lifts explosively. On all other exercises lift the weight as explosively as possible to complete the required number of repetitions in the specified time.

Rest   Take 2:30 between total-body sets and exercises and 2:00 between all other sets and exercises.

Sets and Reps

Week	Power
1	TB = 4 × 2 TL = 3 × 5 @ 9 sec
2	TB = 4 × 3 TL = 3 × 3 @ 5 sec
3	TB = 4 × 2 TL = 3 × 5 @ 9 sec
4	TB = 4 × 3 TL = 3 × 3 @ 5 sec
5	TB = 4 × 2 TL = 3 × 5 @ 9 sec

	Week 1	Week 2	Week 3	Week 4	Week 5
PLYOMETRIC					
Lateral box jump	3 × 6	3 × 6	3 × 6	3 × 6	3 × 6
Reps completed					
TOTAL BODY					
Power snatch TB	4 × 2	4 × 3	4 × 2	4 × 3	4 × 2
Weight lifted					
LOWER BODY					
One-leg squat TL	3 × 5 @ 9 sec	3 × 3 @ 5 sec	3 × 5 @ 9 sec	3 × 3 @ 5 sec	3 × 5 @ 9 sec
Weight lifted					
Lateral squat TL	3 × 5 @ 9 sec	3 × 3 @ 5 sec	3 × 5 @ 9 sec	3 × 3 @ 5 sec	3 × 5 @ 9 sec
Weight lifted					
TRUNK					
Toe touch	3 × 25	3 × 25	3 × 25	3 × 25	3 × 25
Weight lifted					
UPPER BODY					
Incline press TL	3 × 5 @ 9 sec	3 × 3 @ 5 sec	3 × 5 @ 9 sec	3 × 3 @ 5 sec	3 × 5 @ 9 sec
Weight lifted					

Power and Endurance Cycle

Monday

Length 5 weeks

Goals Increase power and muscular endurance.

Intensity Power: Complete the full number of required repetitions on the first set only. Endurance: Complete the full number of required repetitions on each set.

Pace Power: Perform total-body lifts explosively. In all other exercises, lift at a pace that allows completion of the required number of repetitions in the specified time. Endurance: Perform total-body lifts explosively. In all other exercises lift as explosively as possible and lower in three seconds.

Rest Power: Take 2:45 between all sets and exercises. Endurance: Take 1:30 between total-body exercise sets and 1:15 between all other sets and exercises.

Sets and Reps

Week	Power	Endurance
1	TB = 4 × 2 TL = 4 × 3 @ 4 sec	TB = 4 × 6 CL = 4 × 10
2	TB = 4 × 3 TL = 4 × 5 @ 6 sec	TB = 4 × 4 CL = 4 × 8
3	TB = 4 × 2 TL = 4 × 3 @ 4 sec	TB = 4 × 6 CL = 4 × 10
4	TB = 4 × 3 TL = 4 × 5 @ 6 sec	TB = 4 × 4 CL = 4 × 8
5	TB = 4 × 2 TL = 4 × 3 @ 4 sec	TB = 4 × 6 CL = 4 × 10

Endurance: Perform full reps in each set.

	Week 1	Week 2	Week 3	Week 4	Week 5
TOTAL BODY					
Alt power jerk TB	4 × 6	4 × 4	4 × 6	4 × 4	4 × 6
Weight lifted					
LOWER BODY					
One-leg squat CL	4 × 10	4 × 8	4 × 10	4 × 8	4 × 10
Weight lifted					
Side lunge CL	4 × 10	4 × 8	4 × 10	4 × 8	4 × 10
Weight lifted					
TRUNK					
Twisting crunch	3 × 10	3 × 10	3 × 10	3 × 10	3 × 10
Weight lifted					
Twisting back extension	3 × 10	3 × 10	3 × 10	3 × 10	3 × 10
Weight lifted					
UPPER BACK					
Row CL	4 × 10	4 × 8	4 × 10	4 × 8	4 × 10
Weight lifted					

(continued)

Power and Endurance Cycle *(continued)*

Wednesday

Length   4.5 weeks

Goals   Increase power and muscular endurance.

Intensity   Power: Complete the full number of required repetitions on the first set only. Endurance: Complete the full number of required repetitions on each set.

Pace   Power: Perform total-body lifts explosively. In all other exercises lift at a pace that allows completion of the required number of repetitions in the specified time. Endurance: Perform total-body lifts explosively. In all other exercises lift as explosively as possible and lower in 3 seconds.

Rest   Power: Take 2:45 between all sets and exercises. Endurance: Take 1:30 between total-body exercise sets and 1:15 between all other sets and exercises.

Sets and Reps

Week	Power	Endurance
1	TB = 4 × 2 TL = 4 × 3 @ 4 sec	TB = 4 × 6 CL = 4 × 10
2	TB = 4 × 3 TL = 4 × 5 @ 6 sec	TB = 4 × 4 CL = 4 × 8
3	TB = 4 × 2 TL = 4 × 3 @ 4 sec	TB = 4 × 6 CL = 4 × 10
4	TB = 4 × 3 TL = 4 × 5 @ 6 sec	TB = 4 × 4 CL = 4 × 8
5	TB = 4 × 2 TL = 4 × 3 @ 4 sec	TB = 4 × 6 CL = 4 × 10

Power: Complete full reps on first set only.

	Week 1	Week 2	Week 3	Week 4	Week 5
TOTAL BODY					
Clean TB	4 × 2	4 × 3	4 × 2	4 × 3	4 × 2
Weight lifted					
Drop jump and box jump	3 × 5	3 × 5	3 × 5	3 × 5	3 × 5
Reps completed					
LOWER BODY					
Front squat TL	4 × 3 @ 4 sec	4 × 5 @ 6 sec	4 × 3 @ 4 sec	4 × 5 @ 6 sec	4 × 3 @ 4 sec
Weight lifted					
SLDL TL	4 × 3 @ 4 sec	4 × 5 @ 6 sec	4 × 3 @ 4 sec	4 × 5 @ 6 sec	4 × 3 @ 4 sec
Weight lifted					
TRUNK					
Seated twist	3 × 10	3 × 10	3 × 10	3 × 10	3 × 10
Weight lifted					
CHEST					
Incline press TL	4 × 3 @ 4 sec	4 × 5 @ 6 sec	4 × 3 @ 4 sec	4 × 5 @ 6 sec	4 × 3 @ 4 sec
Weight lifted					
Complex: MB lying chest pass	3 × 6	3 × 6	3 × 6	3 × 6	3 × 6
Reps completed					

Friday

Length   4.5 weeks

Goals   Increase power and muscular endurance.

Intensity   Power: Complete the full number of required repetitions on the first set only. Endurance: Complete the full number of required repetitions on each set.

Pace   Power: Perform total-body lifts explosively. In all other exercises lift at a pace that allows completion of the required number of repetitions in the specified time. Endurance: Perform total-body lifts explosively. In all other exercises lift as explosively as possible and lower in 3 seconds

Rest   Power: Take 2:45 between all sets and exercises. Endurance: Take 1:30 between total-body exercise sets and 1:15 between all other sets and exercises.

Sets and Reps

Week	Power	Endurance
1	TB = 4 × 2 TL = 4 × 3 @ 4 sec	TB = 4 × 6 CL = 4 × 10
2	TB = 4 × 3 TL = 4 × 5 @ 6 sec	TB = 4 × 4 CL = 4 × 8
3	TB = 4 × 2 TL = 4 × 3 @ 4 sec	TB = 4 × 6 CL = 4 × 10
4	TB = 4 × 3 TL = 4 × 5 @ 6 sec	TB = 4 × 4 CL = 4 × 8
5	TB = 4 × 2 TL = 4 × 3 @ 4 sec	TB = 4 × 6 CL = 4 × 10

Power: Complete full reps on the first set only.

	Week 1	Week 2	Week 3	Week 4	Week 5
TOTAL BODY					
Alt power clean TB	4 × 2	4 × 3	4 × 2	4 × 3	4 × 2
Weight lifted					
Complex: lateral drop jump and lateral box jump	3 × 5	3 × 5	3 × 5	3 × 5	3 × 5
Reps completed					
CHEST					
Alt bench press TL	4 × 3 @ 4 sec	4 × 5 @ 6 sec	4 × 3 @ 4 sec	4 × 5 @ 6 sec	4 × 3 @ 4 sec
Weight lifted					
Alt incline press TL	4 × 3 @ 4 sec	4 × 5 @ 6 sec	4 × 3 @ 4 sec	4 × 5 @ 6 sec	4 × 3 @ 4 sec
Weight lifted					
TRUNK					
Alt toe touch	3 × 10	3 × 10	3 × 10	3 × 10	3 × 10
Weight lifted					
Back extension	3 × 10	3 × 10	3 × 10	3 × 10	3 × 10
Weight lifted					
SHOULDERS					
Alt shoulder press TL	4 × 3 @ 4 sec	4 × 5 @ 6 sec	4 × 3 @ 4 sec	4 × 5 @ 6 sec	4 × 3 @ 4 sec
Weight lifted					

CHAPTER 10

Training for Power Sports

In the previous chapter, we defined power as work divided by time or as force multiplied by velocity and explained how to manipulate the training variables (e.g., rest times, sets, repetitions) to meet the goal of training to increase power. We also stressed the importance of training for power to improve athletic performance.

In this chapter we look at training for power to improve performance in sports such as the throwing events in track and field and in basketball, volleyball, and softball. Although these sports are different from each, power is important to improving performance in each of them. And because of the relationship between strength and power, well-developed muscular strength is required for optimal performance. Therefore, athletes need to manipulate the training variables to increase both power and strength simultaneously.

In the previous chapter we established that training for power typically includes one to six repetitions with rests of 2:00 to 3:00 minutes between sets and exercises. These variables are further refined to address the endurance needs in particular sports. For example, endurance demands are greater in basketball and volleyball than they are in the throwing events in track and field or softball. The program must be based on the demands of the sport. Throwers and softball players (excluding the pitchers, who require more muscular endurance than do the field players) perform just one to four repetitions of the total-body exercises to allow a greater training load. And basketball and volleyball players perform four to six repetitions to place greater emphasis on muscular endurance. Similarly, the rest periods are be 2:30 to 3:00 or longer for the throwers and the softball players to allow fuller recovery between sets, while the rest periods of 1:30 to 2:00 better focus on muscular endurance for the basketball and volleyball players.

Another variable within your training program is the resistance used. The training percentage applied should be 70 to 100 percent of the single-repetition max for throwers in order to best match the demands of throwing a weighted implement. Greater training loads are required to develop force generation when training to enhance both power and strength. In contrast, the percentages could be lower for basketball players (70-90%) and the volleyball and softball players (60-75%). Training percentages are higher for basketball players than for softball and volleyball players because basketball is a contact sport.

In the previous chapter we also discussed timed exercises that add a time component to the typical set and rep scheme. This shifts the emphasis from how much an athlete can lift to how fast an athlete can lift it. By manipulating the time allowed to complete each repetition, you can increase the emphasis on strength development while also focusing on increasing power. For example, you could write a program requiring four sets of five repetitions, with each set to be completed in eight seconds. This allows the athlete 1.6 seconds to complete each repetition. To place a greater emphasis on force development, you can give the athlete more time to complete each repetition, allowing a heavier training load. So, for example, you could prescribe the same four sets of five repetitions, but allow 13 seconds to complete the set. This increases the time allowed to perform each repetition to 2.6 seconds, which should allow the athlete to use a greater training load.

SAMPLE WORKOUT SCHEDULES

Now that we have a training protocol for power sports that also require high levels of strength, let's look at sample dumbbell workouts that simultaneously develop strength and power. The first workout focuses on power and strength. This workout is suitable for throwers in track and field, who require little muscular endurance because the recovery time available between throws when competing is typically long. The training variables address the goals of developing muscular power and strength. A second sample workout is for basketball players and prioritizes muscular power and strength while also addressing the secondary goal of increasing muscular endurance. The third sample workout is for volleyball players and also focuses on power and strength and endurance. Although sports such as basketball and volleyball are primarily power and strength activities, they also include a muscular endurance component.

Power and Strength Cycle for Throwers

Monday

Length 5 weeks

Goals Increase power and strength.

Intensity On total-body lifts complete the full number of required repetitions on the first set only. On timed exercises complete the full number of repetitions in the specified time.

Pace Perform total-body lifts explosively. On all other exercises lift at a pace that allows completion of the required number of repetitions in the specified time.

Rest Take 2:30 between all sets and exercises.

Sets and Reps

Week	Power and Strength
1	TB = 6 × 2-2-2-1-1-1 CL = 4 × 4 @ 8 sec
2	TB = 5 × 3 CL = 4 × 5 @ 9 sec
3	TB = 6 × 2-2-2-1-1-1 CL = 4 × 4 @ 8 sec
4	TB = 5 × 3 CL = 4 × 5 @ 9 sec
5	TB = 6 × 2-2-2-1-1-1 CL = 4 × 4 @ 8 sec

	Week 1	Week 2	Week 3	Week 4	Week 5
TOTAL BODY					
Power snatch TB	6 × 2-2-2-1-1-1	5 × 3	6 × 2-2-2-1-1-1	5 × 3	6 × 2-2-2-1-1-1
Weight lifted					
Split alt- foot snatch TB	6 × 2 @ 90%	5 × 3 @ 80%	6 × 2 @ 90%	5 × 3 @ 80%	6 × 2 @ 90%
Weight lifted					
Complex: box jump	3 × 4	3 × 4	3 × 4	3 × 4	3 × 4
Reps completed					
LOWER BODY					
Front squat TL	4 × 4 @ 8 sec	4 × 5 @ 9 sec	4 × 4 @ 8 sec	4 × 5 @ 9 sec	4 × 4 @ 8 sec
Weight lifted					
Side lunge TL	4 × 4 @ 8 sec	4 × 5 @ 9 sec	4 × 4 @ 8 sec	4 × 5 @ 9 sec	4 × 4 @ 8 sec
Weight lifted					
Reps completed					
TRUNK					
Toe touch	3 × 10	3 × 10	3 × 10	3 × 10	3 × 10
Weight lifted					
Back extension	3 × 8	3 × 8	3 × 8	3 × 8	3 × 8
Weight lifted					

Note: The following abbreviations are used in the workout tables. TB = total body, one of the Olympic-style lifts or related training exercise; CL = core lift, a multijoint exercise such as a squat; TL = timed lift, the athlete completes the required reps in a specified time; WT = weighted, the exercise uses external resistance to increase training intensity; MB = medicine ball, the exercise is performed with a medicine ball (medicine balls are often used in training programs when the goal of training is to develop power, because medicine balls are designed to be thrown explosively).

(continued)

Power and Strength Cycle for Throwers *(continued)*

Wednesday

Length   5 weeks

Goals   Increase power and strength.

Intensity   On total-body lifts complete the full number of required repetitions on the first set only. On timed exercises complete the full number of required repetitions in the specified time.

Pace   Perform total-body lifts explosively. On all other exercises lift at a pace that allows completion of the required number of repetitions in the specified time.

Rest   Take 2:30 between all sets and exercises.

Sets and Reps

Week	Power and strength
1	TB = 6 × 2 @ 90% TL = 4 × 4 @ 8 sec
2	TB = 5 × 3 @ 80% TL = 4 × 5 @ 9 sec
3	TB = 6 × 2 @ 90% TL = 4 × 4 @ 8 sec
4	TB = 5 × 3 @ 80% TL = 4 × 5 @ 9 sec
5	TB = 6 × 2 @ 90% TL = 4 × 4 @ 8 sec

	Week 1	Week 2	Week 3	Week 4	Week 5
TOTAL BODY					
Alt power jerk TB	3 × 2 @ 75%	3 × 3 @ 70%	3 × 2 @ 75%	3 × 3 @ 70%	3 × 2 @ 75%
Weight lifted (shin)					
Split alt-feet jerk TB	6 × 2 @ 90%	5 × 3 @ 80%	6 × 2 @ 90%	5 × 3 @ 80%	6 × 2 @ 90%
Weight lifted					
LOWER BODY					
Jump squat TL	4 × 4 @ 8 sec	4 × 5 @ 9 sec	4 × 4 @ 8 sec	4 × 5 @ 9 sec	4 × 4 @ 8 sec
Weight lifted					
One-leg squat TL	4 × 4 @ 8 sec	4 × 5 @ 9 sec	4 × 4 @ 8 sec	4 × 5 @ 9 sec	4 × 4 @ 8 sec
Weight lifted (each leg)					
Straight-leg deadlift TL	4 × 4 @ 8 sec	4 × 5 @ 9 sec	4 × 4 @ 8 sec	4 × 5 @ 9 sec	4 × 4 @ 8 sec
Weight lifted					
TRUNK					
Twisting crunch	3 × 10	3 × 10	3 × 10	3 × 10	3 × 10
Weight lifted					
V-up	3 × 10	3 × 10	3 × 10	3 × 10	3 × 10
Weight lifted					
CHEST					
Alt bench press CL	4 × 4 @ 8 sec	4 × 5 @ 9 sec	4 × 4 @ 8 sec	4 × 5 @ 9 sec	4 × 4 @ 8 sec
Weight lifted (total)					

Friday

Length 5 weeks

Goals Increase power and strength.

Intensity On total-body lifts complete the full number of required repetitions on the first set only. On timed exercises complete the full number of required repetitions in the specified time.

Pace Perform total-body lifts explosively. On all other exercises lift at a pace that allows completion of the required number of repetitions in the specified time.

Rest Take 2:30 between all sets and exercises.

Sets and Reps

Week	Power and strength
1	TB = 6 × 2 @ 90% TL = 4 × 4 @ 8 sec
2	TB = 5 × 3 @ 80% TL = 4 × 5 @ 9 sec
3	TB = 6 × 2 @ 90% TL = 4 × 4 @ 8 sec
4	TB = 5 × 3 @ 80% TL = 4 × 5 @ 9 sec
5	TB = 6 × 2 @ 90% TL = 4 × 4 @ 8 sec

	Week 1	Week 2	Week 3	Week 4	Week 5
TOTAL BODY					
Hang power clean TB	3 × 2 @ 75%	3 × 3 @ 70%	3 × 2 @ 75%	3 × 3 @ 70%	3 × 2 @ 75%
Weight lifted					
Clean TB	6 × 2 @ 90%	5 × 3 @ 80%	6 × 2 @ 90%	5 × 3 @ 80%	6 × 2 @ 90%
Weight lifted					
Complex: lateral box jump	3 × 4	3 × 4	3 × 4	3 × 4	3 × 4
Reps completed					
CHEST					
Incline press TL	4 × 4 @ 8 sec	4 × 5 @ 9 sec	4 × 4 @ 8 sec	4 × 5 @ 9 sec	4 × 4 @ 8 sec
Weight lifted					
Complex: MB lying chest pass	3 × 6	3 × 6	3 × 6	3 × 6	3 × 8
Reps completed					
TRUNK					
V-up	3 × 8	3 × 8	3 × 8	3 × 8	3 × 10
Weight lifted					
UPPER BACK					
Row TL	4 × 4 @ 8 sec	4 × 5 @ 9 sec	4 × 4 @ 8 sec	4 × 5 @ 9 sec	4 × 4 @ 8 sec
Weight lifted					

The workouts that follow focus on two physiological goals. The primary goal is increases in power and strength. The secondary goal is to increase muscular endurance.

Power and Strength Cycle for Basketball Players

Monday

Length 5 weeks

Goals Increase power and strength.

Intensity On total-body lifts complete the full number of required repetitions on each set. On timed exercises complete the full number of required repetitions in the specified time period.

Pace Perform total-body lifts explosively. On all other exercises lift at a pace that allows completion of the required number of repetitions in the specified time.

Rest Take 2:00 between total-body sets and exercises and 1:30 between all other sets and exercises.

Sets and Reps

Week	Power and strength
1	TB = 5 × 3 @ 85% TL = 4 × 8 @ 12 sec
2	TB = 5 × 5 @ 80% TL = 4 × 6 @ 10 sec
3	TB = 5 × 3 @ 85% TL = 4 × 8 @ 12 sec
4	TB = 5 × 5 @ 80% TL = 4 × 6 @ 10 sec
5	TB = 5 × 3 @ 85% TL = 4 × 8 @ 12 sec

	Week 1	Week 2	Week 3	Week 4	Week 5
TOTAL BODY					
Power snatch TB	3 × 3 @ 75%	3 × 5 @ 70%	3 × 3 @ 75%	3 × 5 @ 70%	3 × 3 @ 75%
Weight lifted					
Split alt-foot snatch TB	5 × 3 @ 85%	5 × 5 @ 80%	5 × 3 @ 85%	5 × 5 @ 80%	5 × 3 @ 85%
Weight lifted					
Complex: box jump	3 × 4	3 × 4	3 × 4	3 × 4	3 × 4
Reps completed					
LOWER BODY					
Front squat TL	4 × 8 @ 12 sec	4 × 6 @ 10 sec	4 × 8 @ 12 sec	4 × 6 @ 10 sec	4 × 8 @ 12 sec, 4 × 3 @ 5 sec
Weight lifted					
Side lunge TL	4 × 8 @ 12 sec	4 × 6 @ 10 sec	4 × 8 @ 12 sec	4 × 6 @ 10 sec	4 × 8 @ 12 sec, 4 × 3 @ 5 sec
Weight lifted					
TRUNK					
Toe touch	3 × 15	3 × 15	3 × 15	3 × 15	3 × 15
Weight lifted					
Back extension	3 × 12	3 × 12	3 × 12	3 × 12	3 × 12
Weight lifted					

Wednesday (Endurance)

Length 5 weeks

Goals Increase muscular endurance.

Intensity Complete the full number of required repetitions on each set.

Pace Perform total-body lifts explosively. On all other exercises lift as explosively as possible and lower in 2 seconds.

Rest Take 1:30 between total body exercise sets and 1:00 between all other sets and exercises.

Sets and Reps

Week	Endurance*
1	TB = 5 × 6 @ 70% TL = 4 × 10 @ 20 sec
2	TB = 5 × 4 @ 75% TL = 4 × 8 @ 13 sec
3	TB = 5 × 6 @ 70% TL = 4 × 10 @ 20 sec
4	TB = 5 × 4 @ 75% TL = 4 × 8 @ 13 sec
5	TB = 5 × 6 @ 70% TL = 4 × 10 @ 20 sec (2)

*Endurance. Perform full reps during each set.

	Week 1	Week 2	Week 3	Week 4	Week 5
TOTAL BODY					
Alt power snatch TB	3 × 6 @ 70%	3 × 4 @ 75%	3 × 6 @ 70%	3 × 4 @ 75%	3 × 6 @ 70%
Weight lifted					
Split alt-feet snatch TB	5 × 6 @ 77%	5 × 4 @ 82%	5 × 6 @ 77%	5 × 4 @ 82%	5 × 6 @ 77%
Weight lifted					
LOWER BODY					
Jump squat TL	4 × 10 @ 20 sec	4 × 8 @ 13 sec	4 × 10 @ 20 sec	4 × 8 @ 13 sec	4 × 10 @ 20 sec
Weight lifted					
One-leg squat TL	4 × 10 @ 20 sec	4 × 8 @ 13 sec	4 × 10 @ 20 sec	4 × 8 @ 13 sec	4 × 10 @ 20 sec
Weight lifted (each leg)					
Straight-leg deadlift TL	4 × 10 @ 20 sec	4 × 8 @ 13 sec	4 × 10 @ 20 sec	4 × 8 @ 13 sec	4 × 10 @ 20 sec
Weight lifted					
TRUNK					
Twisting crunch	3 × 20	3 × 20	3 × 20	3 × 20	3 × 20
Weight lifted					
V-up	3 × 20	3 × 20	3 × 20	3 × 20	3 × 20
Weight lifted					
CHEST					
Alt bench press CL	4 × 8	4 × 6	4 × 8	4 × 6	4 × 8
Weight lifted (total)					

(continued)

Power and Strength Cycle for Basketball Players *(continued)*

Friday

Length 5 weeks

Goals Increase power and strength.

Intensity On total-body lifts complete the full number of required repetitions on the first set only. On timed exercises complete the full number of required repetitions in the specified time.

Pace Perform total-body lifts explosively. On all other exercises lift at a pace that allows completion of the required number of repetitions in the specified time.

Rest Take 2:00 between total-body sets and exercises and 1:30 between all other sets and exercises.

Sets and Reps

Week	Power and strength
1	TB = 5 × 3 TL = 4 × 8 @ 12 sec
2	TB = 5 × 5 TL = 4 × 6 @ 10 sec
3	TB = 5 × 3 TL = 4 × 8 @ 12 sec
4	TB = 5 × 5 TL = 4 × 6 @ 10 sec
5	TB = 5 × 3 TL = 4 × 8 @ 12 sec

	Week 1	Week 2	Week 3	Week 4	Week 5
TOTAL BODY					
Hang power clean TB	3 × 3 @ 75%	3 × 5 @ 70%	3 × 3 @ 75%	3 × 5 @ 70%	3 × 3 @ 75%
Weight lifted					
Clean TB	5 × 3 @ 85%	5 × 5 @ 80%	5 × 3 @ 85%	5 × 5 @ 80%	5 × 3 @ 85%
Weight lifted					
Complex: lateral box jump	3 × 4	3 × 4	3 × 4	3 × 4	3 × 4
Reps completed					
CHEST					
Incline press TL	4 × 8 @ 12 sec	4 × 6 @ 10 sec	4 × 8 @ 12 sec	4 × 6 @ 10 sec	4 × 8 @ 12 sec
Weight lifted					
Complex: MB lying chest pass	3 × 6	3 × 6	3 × 6	3 × 6	3 × 6
Reps completed					
TRUNK					
V-up	3 × 8	3 × 8	3 × 8	3 × 8	3 × 8
Weight lifted					
UPPER BACK					
Row TL	4 × 8 @ 12 sec	4 × 6 @ 10 sec	4 × 8 @ 12 sec	4 × 6 @ 10 sec	4 × 8 @ 12 sec, 4 × 3 @ 5 sec
Weight lifted					

Power and Strength Cycle for Volleyball Players

Monday

Length 4 weeks

Goal Increase power because of the positive relationship between power and performance.

Intensity Complete the full number of repetitions in good form on the first set only before increasing resistance.

Pace Perform total-body lifts as explosively as possible. Perform timed lifts at a pace that allows completion of the required number of repetitions in the specified time.

Rest Take 2:00 between all sets and exercises.

Sets and Reps

Week	Power and strength
1	TB = 3 × 4 @ 70% TL = 3 × 6 @ 9 sec
2	TB = 3 × 2 @ 75% TL = 3 × 4 @ 8 sec
3	TB = 3 × 4 @ 70% TL = 3 × 6 @ 9 sec
4	TB = 3 × 2 @ 75% TL = 3 × 4 @ 8 sec

	Week 1	Week 2	Week 3	Week 4
TOTAL BODY				
Hang power clean TB	3 × 4 @ 70%	3 × 2 @ 75%	3 × 4 @ 70%	3 × 2 @ 75%
Weight lifted				
Hang clean TB	3 × 4 @ 75%	3 × 2 @ 80%	3 × 4 @ 75%	3 × 2 @ 80%
Weight lifted				
LOWER BODY				
Jump squat TL	2 × 6 @ 9 sec	2 × 4 @ 8 sec	2 × 6 @ 9 sec	2 × 4 @ 8 sec
Weight lifted				
Side lunge TL	3 × 6 @ 9 sec	3 × 4 @ 8 sec	3 × 6 @ 9 sec	3 × 4 @ 8 sec
Weight lifted (total)				
TRUNK				
Twist crunch	3 × 10	3 × 10	3 × 10	3 × 10
Weight lifted				
Back extension	3 × 8	3 × 8	3 × 8	3 × 8
Weight lifted				
UPPER BACK				
Bent row TL	3 × 6 @ 9 sec	3 × 4 @ 8 sec	3 × 6 @ 9 sec	3 × 4 @ 8 sec
Weight lifted				
ROTATOR CUFF				
Internal rotation	2 × 12	2 × 12	2 × 12	2 × 12
Weight lifted				

(continued)

Power and Strength Cycle for Volleyball Players *(continued)*

Wednesday (Endurance)

<u>Length</u> 4 weeks

<u>Goal</u> Increase muscular endurance.

<u>Intensity</u> Complete the full number of repetitions in good form on each set before increasing resistance.

<u>Pace</u> Perform total-body lifts as explosively as possible. Perform timed lifts at a pace that allows completion of the required number of repetitions in the specified time.

<u>Rest</u> Take 1:30 between total-body sets and exercises and 1:00 between all other sets and exercises.

Sets and Reps

Week	Endurance
1	TB = 3 × 3 @ 85% TL = 3 × 8 @ 16 sec
2	TB = 3 × 5 @ 80% TL = 3 × 10 @ 17 sec
3	TB = 3 × 3 @ 85% TL = 3 × 8 @ 16 sec
4	TB = 3 × 5 @ 80% TL = 3 × 10 @ 17 sec

	Week 1	Week 2	Week 3	Week 4
TOTAL BODY				
Power snatch TB	3 × 3 @ 85%	3 × 5 @ 80%	3 × 3 @ 85%	3 × 5 @ 80%
Weight lifted				
Split alt-feet alt snatch TB	3 × 3 @ 87%	3 × 5 @ 82%	3 × 3 @ 87%	3 × 5 @ 82%
Weight lifted				
LOWER BODY				
Jump squat TL	3 × 8 @ 16 sec	3 × 10 @ 17 sec	3 × 8 @ 16 sec	3 × 10 @ 17 sec
Weight lifted				
Arc lunge TL	3 × 8 @ 16 sec	3 × 10 @ 17 sec	3 × 8 @ 16 sec	3 × 10 @ 17 sec
Weight lifted (total)				
TRUNK				
Alt V-up	3 × 10	3 × 10	3 × 10	3 × 10
Weight lifted				
WT back extension	3 × 8	3 × 8	3 × 8	3 × 8
Weight lifted				
CHEST AND SHOULDER				
Alt bench press	3 × 8 @ 16 sec	3 × 10 @ 17 sec	3 × 8 @ 16 sec	3 × 10 @ 17 sec
Weight lifted (total)				
ROTATOR CUFF				
Empty can	2 × 10	2 × 10	2 × 10	2 × 10
Weight lifted				

Friday

Length   4 weeks

Goal   Increase power and strength because of their positive relationship with performance.

Intensity   Complete the full number of repetitions in good form on the first set only before increasing resistance.

Pace   Perform total-body lifts as explosively as possible. Perform timed lifts at a pace that allows completion of the required number of repetitions in the specified time.

Rest   Take 2:00 between all sets and exercises.

Sets and Reps

Week	Power and strength
1	TB = 3 × 4 @ 70% TL = 3 × 6 @ 9 sec
2	TB = 3 × 2 @ 75% TL = 3 × 4 @ 8 sec
3	TB = 3 × 4 @ 70% TL = 3 × 6 @ 9 sec
4	TB = 3 × 2 @ 75% TL = 3 × 4 @ 8 sec

	Week 1	Week 2	Week 3	Week 4
TOTAL BODY				
Power jerk TB	3 × 4 @ 70%	3 × 2 @ 75%	3 × 4 @ 70%	3 × 2 @ 75%
Weight lifted				
Split alt-foot alt jerk TB	3 × 4 @ 75%	3 × 2 @ 80%	3 × 4 @ 75%	3 × 2 @ 80%
Weight lifted				
CHEST				
Bench press TL	4 × 4 @ 5 sec	3 × 6 @ 9 sec	3 × 4 @ 5 sec	3 × 6 @ 9 sec
Weight lifted				
Pullover TL	3 × 4 @ 5 sec	3 × 6 @ 9 sec	3 × 4 @ 5 sec	3 × 6 @ 9 sec
Weight lifted				
TRUNK				
Alt toe touch	3 × 10	3 × 10	3 × 10	3 × 10
Reps completed				
SHOULDERS				
Shoulder press TL	3 × 4 @ 5 sec	3 × 6 @ 9 sec	3 × 4 @ 5 sec	3 × 6 @ 9 sec
Weight lifted (total)				
ROTATOR CUFF				
Functional rotation	2 × 12	2 × 12	2 × 12	2 × 12
Weight lifted				

CHAPTER 11

Training for Speed Sports

Although success in sprint events requires strength, the greater need is speed. So we will explore how to develop the speed required in sports such as the sprint events in track, swimming, and cycling and in short-track speed skating. Although high performance in these sports requires strength, the need is less than it is in football, rugby, and the throwing events in track and field. The greater need is to produce high-velocity movement.

Training to achieve high-velocity movement is primarily a matter of adjusting the training load. Whereas training loads of 70 to 100 percent of one-repetition maximum (1RM) are suggested to increase force generation, the opposite approach is recommended for increasing speed. Speed training programs should use loads of 45 to 70 percent of 1RM. These lighter loads shift the emphasis to training velocity rather than training load.

However, before athletes can train for velocity, they need to develop their force-generation capabilities. Sprinters cannot focus only on speed training; they need to develop a strength base before shifting to high-velocity training. Propelling the body down the track or through the water at maximal speed requires a strength base before shifting the emphasis to speed.

Timed lifts, discussed in chapters 9 and 10, are an important component of speed training. In the example in the chapter on training for power sports, an athlete performs four sets of five repetitions, completing a set in 13 seconds, which allows 2.6 seconds for each repetition. When training for speed sports, a sprinter could perform the same four sets of five repetitions but shorten the time to complete a set to six seconds. This allows just 1.2 seconds per repetition, which focuses on speed rather than force.

Determining how much rest to take between sets and exercises and deciding how many repetitions to perform in set depends on the event the athlete is training for. There are significant differences between the sprint events in track, swimming, skating, and cycling. For example, the world record for the 100-meter freestyle in long-course swimming for men is 46.91, for women it is 52.07. The record for 500 meters in short-track speed skating is 39.937 seconds for men and 42.609 seconds for women. In cycling, the world record for men in the flying 500-meter time trial is

24.758, and for women it is 29.655. In contrast, the world record for the 100 meters on the track for men is 9.58 and 10.49 for women. Although all of these are considered sprint events, the swimmers, cyclists, and skaters have a greater need for endurance than the track sprinters do. This is addressed by manipulating both rest times and the number of repetitions per set. Because the sprint races take longer in swimming, cycling, and short-track speed skating than they do in the 100 meters in track, the rest times between sets and exercises are shorter and the number of repetitions is higher to reflect the need for endurance in these events.

SAMPLE WORKOUT SCHEDULES

The first sample workout is for a track sprinter. The rest times are long and the number of repetitions low to reflect the short duration of this event. This allows a greater emphasis on developing strength and power to better match the demands of the sport.

The second sample workout is for a sprint swimmer. Because of the demands of the sport, the training variables emphasize endurance, which comes into play more than it does for the 100-meter sprinter on the track. We have decreased the rest times and increased the number of repetitions. In addition, we have included compound exercises, which combine two exercises into one, such as a dumbbell front squat to power jerk. Compound exercises increase the duration of each repetition, which develops endurance.

Because water provides greater resistance than air does, a training program for swimmers focuses on increasing and maintaining strength. This occurs primarily by increasing the percentage of 1RM used when performing total-body exercises and by increasing the time allowed to complete each repetition during timed exercises.

The third sample workout is for a cyclist competing in the longer sprint events. Because of the length of these races, we have adjusted the training variables to emphasize endurance. We have reduced the rest times and increased the number of repetitions. Compound exercises develop muscular endurance.

A final example workout is provided for short track speed skating. Again, the rest times are brief, the repetitions are at a higher range, and compound exercises are used in conjunction with the weightlifting movements, timed exercises, and plyometric activities to meet the needs of power, speed, and muscular endurance.

Power Cycle for Track Sprinters

Monday

Length   5 weeks

Goals   Increase power and strength because of the relationship between power, strength, and speed.

Intensity   On total-body lifts complete the full number of repetitions on the first set only. On timed exercises complete the full number of required repetitions in the specified time.

Pace   Perform total-body lifts explosively. On all other exercises lift at a pace that allows completion of the required number of repetitions in the specified time.

Rest   Take 3:00 between all sets and exercises.

Sets and Reps

Week	Power cycle
1	TB = 6 × 3 @ 50-55% TL = 4 × 6 @ 9 sec
2	TB = 5 × 2 @ 60-65% TL = 4 × 3 @ 4 sec
3	TB = 6 × 3 @ 50-55% TL = 4 × 6 @ 9 sec
4	TB = 5 × 2 @ 60-65% TL = 4 × 3 @ 4 sec
5	TB = 6 × 3 @ 50-55% TL = 4 × 6 @ 9 sec

	Week 1	Week 2	Week 3	Week 4	Week 5
TOTAL BODY					
Alt power jerk TB	6 × 3 @ 50%	5 × 2 @ 60%	6 × 3 @ 50%	5 × 2 @ 60%	6 × 3 @ 50%
Weight lifted					
Complex: depth jump	4 × 5	4 × 5	4 × 5	4 × 5	4 × 5
Reps completed					
Complex: split alt-foot alt jerk TB	6 × 3 @ 55%	5 × 2 @ 65%	6 × 3 @ 55%	5 × 2 @ 65%	6 × 3 @ 55%
Weight lifted					
Complex: squat jump	4 × 5	4 × 5	4 × 5	4 × 5	4 × 5
Reps completed					
LOWER BODY					
Jump squat TL	4 × 6 @ 9 sec	4 × 3 @ 4 sec	4 × 6 @ 9 sec	4 × 3 @ 4 sec	4 × 6 @ 9 sec
Weight lifted					
Straight-leg deadlift TL	4 × 6 @ 9 sec	4 × 3 @ 4 sec	4 × 6 @ 9 sec	4 × 3 @ 4 sec	4 × 6 @ 9 sec
Weight lifted					
TRUNK					
Twisting crunch	3 × 10	3 × 10	3 × 10	3 × 10	3 × 10
Weight lifted					
UPPER BACK					
Row TL	4 × 6 @ 9 sec	4 × 3 @ 4 sec	4 × 6 @ 9 sec	4 × 3 @ 4 sec	4 × 6 @ 9 sec
Reps completed					

Note: The following abbreviations are used in the workout tables. TB = total body, one of the Olympic-style lifts or related training exercise; CL = core lift, a multijoint exercise such as a squat; TL = timed lift, the athlete completes the required reps in a specified time; AL = auxiliary lift, a single-joint exercise such as a biceps curl; MB = medicine ball, the exercise is performed with a medicine ball (medicine balls are often used in training programs when the goal of training is to develop power, because medicine balls are designed to be thrown explosively)

(continued)

Power Cycle for Track Sprinters *(continued)*

Wednesday

Length 5 weeks

Goals Increase power and strength because of the relationship between power, strength, and speed.

Intensity On total-body lifts complete the full number of required repetitions on the first set only. On timed exercises complete the full number of required repetitions in the specified time.

Pace Perform total-body lifts explosively. On all other exercises lift at a pace that allows completion of the required number of repetitions in the specified time.

Rest Take 3:00 between all sets and exercises.

Sets and Reps

Week	Power cycle
1	TB = 6 × 3 @ 50-55% TL = 4 × 6 @ 9 sec
2	TB = 5 × 2 @ 60-65% TL = 4 × 3 @ 4 sec
3	TB = 6 × 3 @ 50-55% TL = 4 × 6 @ 9 sec
4	TB = 5 × 2 @ 60-65% TL = 4 × 3 @ 4 sec
5	TB = 6 × 3 @ 50-55% TL = 4 × 6 @ 9 sec

	Week 1	Week 2	Week 3	Week 4	Week 5
TOTAL BODY					
Alt power snatch TB	6 × 3 @ 50%	5 × 2 @ 60%	6 × 3 @ 50%	5 × 2 @ 60%	6 × 3 @ 50%
Weight lifted (shin)					
Complex: pyramid box jump (4 boxes)	4 × 4	4 × 5	4 × 4	4 × 5	4 × 4
Reps completed					
Complex: split alt-feet alt snatch TB	6 × 3 @ 55%	5 × 2 @ 65%	6 × 3 @ 55%	5 × 2 @ 65%	6 × 3 @ 55%
Weight lifted					
Complex: incline rope hop	4 × 5	4 × 5	4 × 5	4 × 5	4 × 5
Reps completed					
LOWER BODY					
Jump split lunge TL	4 × 6 @ 9 sec	4 × 3 @ 4 sec	4 × 6 @ 9 sec	4 × 3 @ 4 sec	4 × 6 @ 9 sec
Weight lifted					
TRUNK					
Press crunch	3 × 10	3 × 10	3 × 10	3 × 10	3 × 10
Weight lifted					
CHEST					
Alt bench press CL	4 × 6 @ 9 sec	4 × 3 @ 4 sec	4 × 6 @ 9 sec	4 × 3 @ 4 sec	4 × 6 @ 9 sec
Weight lifted					

Friday

Length   5 weeks

Goals   Increase power and strength because of the relationship between power, strength, and speed.

Intensity   On total-body lifts complete the full number of required repetitions on the first set only. On timed exercises complete the full number of required repetitions in the specified time.

Pace   Perform total-body lifts explosively. On all other exercises lift at a pace that allows completion of the required number of repetitions in the specified time.

Rest   Take 3:00 between all sets and exercises.

Sets and Reps

Week	Power cycle
1	TB = 6 × 3 @ 50-55% TL = 4 × 6 @ 9 sec
2	TB = 5 × 2 @ 60-65% TL = 4 × 3 @ 4 sec
3	TB = 6 × 3 @ 50-55% TL = 4 × 6 @ 9 sec
4	TB = 5 × 2 @ 60-65% TL = 4 × 3 @ 4 sec
5	TB = 6 × 3 @ 50-55% TL = 4 × 6 @ 9 sec

	Week 1	Week 2	Week 3	Week 4	Week 5
TOTAL BODY					
Alt power clean TB	6 × 3 @ 50%	5 × 2 @ 60%	6 × 3 @ 50%	5 × 2 @ 60%	6 × 3 @ 50%
Weight lifted					
Complex: lateral cone hop	4 × 5	4 × 5	4 × 5	4 × 5	4 × 5
Reps completed					
Complex: alt hang clean TB	6 × 3 @ 55%	5 × 2 @ 65%%	6 × 3 @ 55%	5 × 2 @ 65%	6 × 3 @ 55%
Weight lifted					
Complex: lateral drop jump and lateral box jumps	4 × 5	4 × 5	4 × 5	4 × 5	4 × 5
Reps completed					
CHEST					
Alt incline press TL	4 × 6 @ 9 sec	4 × 3 @ 4 sec	4 × 6 @ 9 sec	4 × 3 @ 4 sec	4 × 6 @ 9 sec
Weight lifted					
Complex: MB lying chest pass	4 × 5	4 × 5	4 × 5	4 × 5	4 × 5
Reps completed					
TRUNK					
V-up	3 × 10	3 × 10	3 × 10	3 × 10	3 × 10
Weight lifted					
UPPER BACK					
Upright row TL	4 × 6 @ 9 sec	4 × 3 @ 4 sec	4 × 6 @ 9 sec	4 × 3 @ 4 sec	4 × 6 @ 9 sec
Weight lifted					

Power Cycle for Swim Sprinters

Monday

Length 5 weeks

Goals Increase power, strength (because of the relationship between power, strength, and speed), and muscular endurance.

Intensity On total-body lifts complete the full number of required repetitions on each set. On timed exercises complete the full number of required repetitions in the specified time.

Pace Perform total-body lifts explosively. On all other exercises lift at a pace that allows completion of the required number of repetitions in the specified time.

Rest Take 1:30 between all sets and exercises.

Sets and Reps

Week	Power cycle
1	TB = 4 × 5 @ 70% TL = 3 × 30 @ 51 sec AL = 3 × 20
2	TB = 4 × 6 @ 65% TL = 3 × 25 @ 40 sec AL = 3 × 20
3	TB = 4 × 5 @ 70% TL = 3 × 30 @ 51 sec AL = 3 × 20
4	TB = 4 × 6 @ 65% TL = 3 × 25 @ 40 sec AL = 3 × 20
5	TB = 4 × 5 @ 70% TL = 3 × 30 @ 51 sec AL = 3 × 20

	Week 1	Week 2	Week 3	Week 4	Week 5
TOTAL BODY					
Front squat to power jerk TB	4 × 5 @ 70%	4 × 6 @ 65%	4 × 5 @ 70%	4 × 6 @ 65%	4 × 5 @ 70%
Weight lifted					
Complex: depth jump	3 × 8	3 × 8	3 × 8	3 × 8	3 × 8
Reps completed					
LOWER BODY					
Jump squat TL	3 × 30 @ 51 sec	3 × 25 @ 40 sec	3 × 30 @ 51 sec	3 × 25 @ 40 sec	3 × 30 @ 51 sec
Weight lifted					
Straight-leg deadlift TL	3 × 30 @ 51 sec	3 × 25 @ 40 sec	3 × 30 @ 51 sec	3 × 25 @ 40 sec	3 × 30 @ 51 sec
Weight lifted					
TRUNK					
V-up	3 × 50	3 × 50	3 × 50	3 × 50	3 × 50
Weight lifted					
UPPER BODY					
Upright row TL	3 × 30 @ 51 sec	3 × 25 @ 40 sec	3 × 30 @ 51 sec	3 × 25 @ 40 sec	3 × 30 @ 51 sec
Weight lifted					
Front raise AL	3 × 20	3 × 20	3 × 20	3 × 20	3 × 20
Weight lifted					
ROTATOR CUFF					
External rotation	2 × 15	2 × 15	2 × 15	2 × 15	2 × 15
Reps completed					

Wednesday

Length 5 weeks

Goals Increase power, strength (because of the relationship between power, strength and speed), and muscular endurance.

Intensity On total-body lifts complete the full number of required repetitions on each set. On timed exercises complete the full number of required repetitions in the specified time.

Pace Perform total-body lifts explosively. On all other exercises lift at a pace that allows completion of the required number of repetitions in the specified time.

Rest Take 1:30 between all sets and exercises.

Sets and Reps

Week	Power cycle
1	TB = 4 × 5 @ 70% TL = 3 × 30 @ 51 sec AL = 3 × 20
2	TB = 4 × 6 @ 65% TL = 3 × 25 @ 40 sec AL = 3 × 20
3	TB = 4 × 5 @ 70% TL = 3 × 30 @ 51 sec AL = 3 × 20
4	TB = 4 × 6 @ 65% TL = 3 × 25 @ 40 sec AL = 3 × 20
5	TB = 4 × 5 @ 70% TL = 3 × 30 @ 51 sec AL = 3 × 20

	Week 1	Week 2	Week 3	Week 4	Week 5
TOTAL BODY					
Squat to alt power snatch to lunge TB	4 × 5 @ 70%	4 × 6 @ 65%	4 × 5 @ 70%	4 × 6 @ 65%	4 × 5 @ 70%
Weight lifted (shin)					
Complex: box jump	3 × 8	3 × 8	3 × 8	3 × 8	3 × 8
Reps completed					
LOWER BODY					
Front squat TL	3 × 30 @ 51 sec	3 × 25 @ 40 sec	3 × 30 @ 51 sec	3 × 25 @ 40 sec	3 × 30 @ 51 sec
Weight lifted					
TRUNK					
Alt press crunch	3 × 50	3 × 50	3 × 50	3 × 50	3 × 50
Weight lifted					
UPPER BODY					
Alt bench press TL	3 × 30 @ 51 sec	3 × 25 @ 40 sec	3 × 30 @ 51 sec	3 × 25 @ 40 sec	3 × 30 @ 51 sec
Weight lifted					
Complex: MB standing pullover pass	3 × 8	3 × 8	3 × 8	3 × 8	3 × 8
Reps completed					
Complex: bent lateral raise AL	3 × 20	3 × 20	3 × 20	3 × 20	3 × 20
Weight lifted					
ROTATOR CUFF					
Internal rotation	2 × 15	2 × 15	2 × 15	2 × 15	2 × 15
Reps completed					

(continued)

Power Cycle for Track Sprinters *(continued)*

Friday

<u>Length</u>   5 weeks

<u>Goals</u>   Increase power, strength (because of the relationship between power, strength and speed), and muscular endurance.

<u>Intensity</u>   On total-body lifts complete the full number of required repetitions on the each set. On timed exercises complete the full number of required repetitions in the specified time.

<u>Pace</u>   Perform total-body lifts explosively. On all other exercises lift at a pace that allows completion of the required number of repetitions in the specified time.

<u>Rest</u>   Take 1:30 between all sets and exercises.

Sets and Reps

Week	Power cycle
1	TB = 4 × 5 @ 70% TL = 3 × 30 @ 51 sec AL = 3 × 20
2	TB = 4 × 6 @ 65% TL = 3 × 25 @ 40 sec AL = 3 × 20
3	TB = 4 × 5 @ 70% TL = 3 × 30 @ 51 sec AL = 3 × 20
4	TB = 4 × 6 @ 65% TL = 3 × 25 @ 40 sec AL = 3 × 20
5	TB = 4 × 5 @ 70% TL = 3 × 30 @ 51 sec AL = 3 × 20

	Week 1	Week 2	Week 3	Week 4	Week 5
TOTAL BODY					
Hang power clean to front squat to power jerk TB	4 × 5 @ 70%	4 × 6 @ 65%	4 × 5 @ 70%	4 × 6 @ 65%	4 × 5 @ 70%
Weight lifted					
Complex: cone hop	3 × 12	3 × 12	3 × 12	3 × 12	3 × 12
Reps complete					
CHEST					
Alt incline press TL	3 × 30 @ 51 sec	3 × 25 @ 40 sec	3 × 30 @ 51 sec	3 × 25 @ 40 sec	3 × 30 @ 51 sec
Weight lifted					
Complex: MB lying chest ball	3 × 12	3 × 12	3 × 12	3 × 12	3 × 12
Reps completed					
TRUNK					
V-up	3 × 30	3 × 30	3 × 30	3 × 30	3 × 30
Weight lifted					
UPPER BACK					
Row TL	3 × 30 @ 51 sec	3 × 25 @ 40 sec	3 × 30 @ 51 sec	3 × 25 @ 40 sec	3 × 30 @ 51 sec
Weight lifted					
Lateral raise AL	3 × 20	3 × 20	3 × 20	3 × 20	3 × 20
Weight lifted					
ROTATOR CUFF					
Empty can	2 × 15	2 × 15	2 × 15	2 × 15	2 × 15
Weight lifted					

Power Cycle for Sprint Cyclists

Monday

Length   5 weeks

Goals   Increase power (because of the relationship between power and speed) and muscular endurance.

Intensity   On total-body lifts complete the full number of required repetitions on each set. On timed exercises complete the full number of required repetitions in the specified time.

Pace   Perform total-body lifts explosively. On all other exercises lift at a pace that allows completion of the required number of repetitions in the specified time.

Rest   Take 1:45 between all sets and exercises.

Sets and Reps

Week	Power cycle
1	TB = 5 × 4 @ 55-60% TL = 4 × 17 @ 23 sec AL = 3 × 10
2	TB = 5 × 6 @ 50-55% TL = 4 × 24 @ 29 sec AL = 3 × 8
3	TB = 5 × 4 @ 55-60% TL = 4 × 17 @ 23 sec AL = 3 × 10
4	TB = 5 × 6 @ 50-55% TL = 4 × 24 @ 29 sec AL = 3 × 8
5	TB = 5 × 4 @ 55-60% TL = 4 × 17 @ 23 sec AL = 3 × 10

	Week 1	Week 2	Week 3	Week 4	Week 5
TOTAL BODY					
Front squat to power jerk TB	5 × 4 @ 55%	5 × 6 @ 50%	5 × 4 @ 55%	5 × 6 @ 50%	5 × 4 @ 55%
Weight lifted					
Complex: single-leg box jump	4 × 6	4 × 6	4 × 6	4 × 6	4 × 6
Reps completed (each leg)					
Complex: split alt-foot alt snatch TB	5 × 4 @ 60%	5 × 3 @ 55%	5 × 4 @ 60%	5 × 3 @ 55%	5 × 4 @ 60%
Weight lifted					
Complex: single-leg squat jump	4 × 6	4 × 6	4 × 6	4 × 6	4 × 6
Reps completed (each leg)					
LOWER BODY					
Single-leg jump squat TL	4 × 17 @ 23 sec	4 × 24 @ 29 sec	4 × 17 @ 23 sec	4 × 24 @ 29 sec	4 × 17 @ 23 sec
Weight lifted (each leg)					
Single-leg straight-leg deadlift TL (each leg)	4 × 17 @ 23 sec	4 × 24 @ 29 sec	4 × 17 @ 23 sec	4 × 24 @ 29 sec	4 × 17 @ 23 sec
Weight lifted					
TRUNK					
Toe touch	3 × 25	3 × 25	3 × 25	3 × 25	3 × 25
Weight lifted					
UPPER BACK					
Upright row AL	3 × 10	3 × 8	3 × 10	3 × 8	3 × 10
Reps completed					

(continued)

Power Cycle for Sprint Cyclists *(continued)*

Wednesday

Length   5 weeks

Goals   Increase power (because of the relationship between power and speed) and muscular endurance.

Intensity   On total-body lifts complete the full number of required repetitions on each set. On timed exercises complete the full number of required repetitions in the specified time.

Pace   Perform total-body lifts explosively. On all other exercises lift at a pace that allows completion of the required number of repetitions in the specified time.

Rest   Take 1:45 between all sets and exercises.

Sets and Reps

Week	Power cycle
1	TB = 5 × 4 @ 55-60% TL = 4 × 17 @ 23 sec
2	TB = 5 × 6 @ 50-55% TL = 4 × 24 @ 29 sec
3	TB = 5 × 4 @ 55-60% TL = 4 × 17 @ 23 sec
4	TB = 5 × 6 @ 50-55% TL = 4 × 24 @ 29 sec
5	TB = 5 × 4 @ 55-60% TL = 4 × 17 @ 23 sec

	Week 1	Week 2	Week 3	Week 4	Week 5
TOTAL BODY					
Squat to alt power snatch TB	5 × 4 @ 55%	5 × 6 @ 50%	5 × 4 @ 55%	5 × 6 @ 50%	5 × 4 @ 55%
Weight lifted (shin)					
Complex: single-leg pyramid box jump (4 boxes)	4 × 6	4 × 6	4 × 6	4 × 6	4 × 6
Reps completed (each leg)					
Complex: hang clean alt-foot alt jerk TB	5 × 4 @ 60%	5 × 3 @ 55%	5 × 4 @ 60%	5 × 3 @ 55%	5 × 4 @ 60%
Weight lifted					
Complex: single-leg incline rope hop	4 × 6	4 × 6	4 × 6	4 × 6	4 × 6
Reps completed					
LOWER BODY					
Jump split lunge TL	4 × 17 @ 23 sec	4 × 24 @ 29 sec	4 × 17 @ 23 sec	4 × 24 @ 29 sec	4 × 17 @ 23 sec
Weight lifted					
TRUNK					
V-up	3 × 25	3 × 25	3 × 25	3 × 25	3 × 25
Weight lifted					
CHEST					
Incline press CL	3 × 10	3 × 8	3 × 10	3 × 8	3 × 10
Weight lifted					

Friday

Length 5 weeks

Goals Increase power (because of the relationship between power and speed) and muscular endurance.

Intensity On total-body lifts complete the full number of required repetitions on the first set only. On timed exercises complete the full number of required repetitions in the specified time.

Pace Perform total-body lifts explosively. On all other exercises lift at a pace that allows completion of the required number of repetitions in the specified time.

Rest Take 1:45 between all sets and exercises.

Sets and Reps

Week	Power cycle
1	TB = 5 × 4 @ 55-60% TL = 4 × 17 @ 23 sec
2	TB = 5 × 6 @ 50-55% TL = 4 × 24 @ 29 sec
3	TB = 5 × 4 @ 55-60% TL = 4 × 17 @ 23 sec
4	TB = 5 × 6 @ 50-55% TL = 4 × 24 @ 29 sec
5	TB = 5 × 4 @ 55-60% TL = 4 × 17 @ 23 sec

	Week 1	Week 2	Week 3	Week 4	Week 5
TOTAL BODY					
Alt power clean to split alt-foot alt power jerk TB	5 × 4 @ 55%	5 × 6 @ 50%	5 × 4 @ 55%	5 × 6 @ 50%	5 × 4 @ 55%
Weight lifted					
Complex: single-leg lateral cone hop	4 × 6	4 × 6	4 × 6	4 × 6	4 × 6
Reps complete (each leg)					
Complex: alt hang clean to alt-foot alt jerk TB	5 × 4 @ 60%	5 × 3 @ 55%	5 × 4 @ 60%	5 × 3 @ 55%	5 × 4 @ 60%
Weight lifted					
Complex: single-leg lateral drop jump and lateral box jump	4 × 6	4 × 6	4 × 6	4 × 6	4 × 6
Reps completed (each leg)					
CHEST					
Bench press TL	4 × 17 @ 23 sec	4 × 24 @ 29 sec	4 × 17 @ 23 sec	4 × 24 @ 29 sec	4 × 17 @ 23 sec
Weight lifted					
TRUNK					
V-up	3 × 25	3 × 25	3 × 25	3 × 25	3 × 25
Weight lifted					
UPPER BACK					
Upright row TL	4 × 17 @ 23 sec	4 × 24 @ 29 sec	4 × 17 @ 23 sec	4 × 24 @ 29 sec	4 × 17 @ 23 sec
Weight lifted					

Power Cycle for Short-Track Speed Skaters

Monday

Length 5 weeks

Goals Increase power (because of the relationship between power and speed) and muscular endurance.

Intensity On total-body lifts complete the full number of required repetitions on each set. On timed exercises complete the full number of required repetitions in the specified time.

Pace Perform total-body lifts explosively. On all other exercises lift at a pace that allows completion of the required number of repetitions in the specified time.

Rest Take 1:40 between all sets and exercises.

Sets and Reps

Week	Power cycle
1	TB = 4 × 4 @ 50-55% TL = 3 × 28 @ 39 sec
2	TB = 4 × 6 @ 45-50% TL = 3 × 25 @ 30 sec
3	TB = 4 × 4 @ 50-55% TL = 3 × 28 @ 39 sec
4	TB = 4 × 6 @ 45-55% TL = 3 × 25 @ 30 sec
5	TB = 4 × 4 @ 50-55% TL = 3 × 28 @ 39 sec

	Week 1	Week 2	Week 3	Week 4	Week 5
TOTAL BODY					
Alt power clean to alt power jerk TB	4 × 4 @ 50-55%	4 × 6 @ 45-50%	4 × 4 @ 50-55%	× 6 @ 45-50%	4 × 4 @ 50-55%
Weight lifted					
Complex: single-leg box jump	4 × 6	4 × 6	4 × 6	4 × 6	4 × 6
Reps completed (each leg)					
Complex: split alt-foot alt jerk TB	4 × 4 @ 50-55%	4 × 6 @ 45-50%	4 × 4 @ 50-55%	4 × 6 @ 45-50%	4 × 4 @ 50-55%
Weight lifted					
Complex: single-leg squat jump	4 × 6	4 × 6	4 × 6	4 × 6	4 × 6
Reps completed (each leg)					
LOWER BODY					
Single-leg jump squat TL	3 × 28 @ 39 sec	3 × 25 @ 30 sec	3 × 28 @ 39 sec	3 × 25 @ 30 sec	3 × 28 @ 39 sec
Weight lifted (each leg)					
Single-leg straight-leg deadlift TL	3 × 28 @ 39 sec	3 × 25 @ 30 sec	3 × 28 @ 39 sec	3 × 25 @ 30 sec	3 × 28 @ 39 sec
Weight lifted (each leg)					
TRUNK					
Twisting crunch	3 × 25	3 × 25	3 × 25	3 × 25	3 × 25
Weight lifted					
UPPER BACK					
Row TL	3 × 28 @ 39 sec	3 × 25 @ 30 sec	3 × 28 @ 39 sec	3 × 25 @ 30 sec	3 × 28 @ 39 sec
Reps completed					

Wednesday

Length 5 weeks

Goals Increase power (because of the relationship between power and speed) and muscular endurance

Intensity On total-body lifts complete the full number of required repetitions on each set. On timed exercises complete the full number of required repetitions in the specified time.

Pace Perform total-body lifts explosively. On all other exercises lift at a pace that allows completion of the required number of repetitions in the specified time.

Rest Take 1:40 between all sets and exercises.

Sets and Reps

Week	Power cycle
1	TB = 4 × 4 @ 50-55% TL = 3 × 28 @ 39 sec
2	TB = 4 × 6 @ 45-50% TL = 3 × 25 @ 30 sec
3	TB = 4 × 4 @ 50-55% TL = 3 × 28 @ 39 sec
4	TB = 4 × 6 @ 45-55% TL = 3 × 25 @ 30 sec
5	TB = 4 × 4 @ 50-55% TL = 3 × 28 @ 39 sec

	Week 1	Week 2	Week 3	Week 4	Week 5
TOTAL BODY					
Squat to alt power snatch TB	4 × 4 @ 50-55%	4 × 6 @ 45-50%	4 × 4 @ 50-55%	4 × 6 @ 45-50%	4 × 4 @ 50-55%
Weight lifted (shin)					
Complex: single-leg pyramid box jump (4 boxes)	4 × 6	4 × 6	4 × 6	4 × 6	4 × 6
Reps completed (each leg)					
Complex: split alt-foot alt snatch TB	4 × 4 @ 50-55%	4 × 6 @ 45-50%	4 × 4 @ 50-55%	4 × 6 @ 45-50%	4 × 4 @ 50-55%
Weight lifted					
Complex: single-leg incline rope hop	4 × 6	4 × 6	4 × 6	4 × 6	4 × 6
Reps completed					
LOWER BODY					
Jump split lunge TL	3 × 28 @ 39 sec	3 × 25 @ 30 sec	3 × 28 @ 39 sec	3 × 25 @ 30 sec	3 × 28 @ 39 sec
Weight lifted					
TRUNK					
Press crunch	3 × 25	3 × 25	3 × 25	3 × 25	3 × 25
Weight lifted					
CHEST					
Alt bench press CL	3 × 28 @ 39 sec	3 × 25 @ 30 sec	3 × 28 @ 39 sec	3 × 25 @ 30 sec	3 × 28 @ 39 sec
Weight lifted					
UPPER BACK					
Bent lateral raise TL	3 × 28 @ 39 sec	3 × 25 @ 30 sec	3 × 28 @ 39 sec	3 × 25 @ 30 sec	3 × 28 @ 39 sec
Weight lifted					

(continued)

Power Cycle for Short-Track Speed Skaters *(continued)*

Friday

Length 5 weeks

Goals Increase power (because of the relationship between power and speed) and muscular endurance.

Intensity On total-body lifts complete the full number of required repetitions on the first set only. On timed exercises complete the full number of required repetitions in the specified time.

Pace Perform total-body lifts explosively. On all other exercises lift at a pace that allows completion of the required number of repetitions in the specified time.

Rest Take 1:40 between all sets and exercises.

Sets and Reps

Week	Power cycle
1	TB = 4 × 4 @ 50-55% TL = 3 × 28 @ 39 sec
2	TB = 4 × 6 @ 45-50% TL = 3 × 25 @ 30 sec
3	TB = 4 × 4 @ 50-55% TL = 3 × 28 @ 39 sec
4	TB = 4 × 6 @ 45-55% TL = 3 × 25 @ 30 sec
5	TB = 4 × 4 @ 50-55% TL = 3 × 28 @ 39 sec

	Week 1	Week 2	Week 3	Week 4	Week 5
TOTAL BODY					
Alt power clean to squat TB	4 × 4 @ 50-55%	4 × 6 @ 45-50%	4 × 4 @ 50-55%	4 × 6 @ 45-50%	4 × 4 @ 50-55%
Weight lifted					
Complex: single-leg lateral cone hop	4 × 6	4 × 6	4 × 6	4 × 6	4 × 6
Reps complete (each leg)					
Complex: alt hang clean TB	4 × 4 @ 50-55%	4 × 6 @ 45-50%	4 × 4 @ 50-55%	4 × 6 @ 45-50%	4 × 4 @ 50-55%
Weight lifted					
Complex: single-leg lateral drop jump and lateral box jump	4 × 6	4 × 6	4 × 6	4 × 6	4 × 6
Reps completed (each leg)					
CHEST					
Alt bench press TL	3 × 28 @ 39 sec	3 × 25 @ 30 sec	3 × 28 @ 39 sec	3 × 25 @ 30 sec	3 × 28 @ 39 sec
Weight lifted					
UPPER BACK					
Upright row TL	3 × 28 @ 39 sec	3 × 25 @ 30 sec	3 × 28 @ 39 sec	3 × 25 @ 30 sec	3 × 28 @ 39 sec
Weight lifted					

CHAPTER 12

Training for Agility and Balance Sports

Dumbbells lend themselves perfectly to balance sports such as wrestling, soccer, ice hockey, and downhill skiing. Although these sports are different from each other, they all require the ability to maintain bodily equilibrium to be able to perform at a high level. Choosing the right dumbbell exercises will not only develop muscle size, strength, power, and endurance but also improve balance.

The focus on balance when using dumbbells is primarily the result of being able to perform both alternating-arm and single-arm movements when training. However, even moving both dumbbells simultaneously contributes more effectively to developing balance because of the need to control two separate implements.

Another advantage of dumbbell training is that it is safer to perform one-leg exercises with dumbbells than to perform the same exercise with a barbell. For example, when performing one-leg squats, it is easier to safely drop the dumbbells to floor than it is to drop a barbell from shoulder height.

SAMPLE WORKOUT SCHEDULES

Because the balance sports mentioned earlier—ice hockey, wrestling, skiing, soccer—have unique demands and requirements, we cannot provide one sample workout that will improve balance in the athletes that participate in these sports. Instead, we include a workout for each sport.

The soccer workout is broken into two schemes, one for field players and one for goalies. Field players require more muscular endurance than goalies do, so their workout calls for more repetitions. Because goalies use quick, explosive movements, their workout focuses on developing strength and power.

Strength Cycle for Wrestlers

Monday

Length   5 weeks

Goal   Increase strength to improve balance and agility.

Intensity   Complete the full number of repetitions on the first set only. Use good form.

Pace   Perform total-body lifts explosively. On all other exercises lift explosively and lower in 2 seconds.

Rest   Take 2:30 between total-body exercises and 2:00 between all other sets and exercises.

Sets and Reps

Week	Strength cycle
1	TB = 5 × 2 CL = 4 × 2 AL = 3 × 5
2	TB = 5 × 4 CL = 4 × 4 AL = 3 × 5
3	TB = 5 × 2 CL = 4 × 2 AL = 3 × 5
4	TB = 5 × 4 CL = 4 × 4 AL = 3 × 5
5	TB = 5 × 2 CL = 4 × 2 AL = 3 × 5

	Week 1	Week 2	Week 3	Week 4	Week 5
TOTAL BODY					
Alt power jerk TB	5 × 2	5 × 4	5 × 2	5 × 4	5 × 2
Weight lifted					
Split alt-foot alt jerk TB	5 × 2	5 × 4	5 × 2	5 × 4	5 × 2
Weight lifted					
LOWER BODY					
One-leg squat CL	4 × 4	4 × 2	4 × 4	4 × 2	4 × 4
Weight lifted					
One-leg straight-leg deadlift CL	4 × 4	4 × 2	4 × 4	4 × 2	4 × 4
Weight lifted					
TRUNK					
Twisting crunch	3 × 12	3 × 12	3 × 12	3 × 12	3 × 12
Weight lifted					
BACK					
Row CL	4 × 4	4 × 2	4 × 4	4 × 2	4 × 4
Weight lifted					
BICEPS					
Alt curls AL	3 × 5	3 × 5	3 × 5	3 × 5	3 × 5
Weight lifted					

Note: The following abbreviations are used in the workout tables. TB = total body, one of the Olympic-style lifts or related training exercise; CL = core lift, a multijoint exercise such as a squat; TL = timed lift, the athlete completes the required reps in a specified time; AL = auxiliary lift, a single-joint exercise such as a biceps curl; a dumbbell; MR = manual resistance, a partner provides resistance.

Tuesday

Length 5 weeks

Goal Increase strength to improve balance and agility.

Intensity Complete the full number of required repetitions on the first set only. Use good form.

Pace Perform total-body lifts explosively. On all other exercises lift explosively and lower in 2 seconds.

Rest Take 2:30 between total-body exercises and 2:00 between all other sets and exercises.

Sets and Reps

Week	Strength cycle
1	TB = 5 × 2 CL = 4 × 2
2	TB = 5 × 4 CL = 4 × 4
3	TB = 5 × 2 CL = 4 × 2
4	TB = 5 × 4 CL = 4 × 4
5	TB = 5 × 2 CL = 4 × 2

	Week 1	Week 2	Week 3	Week 4	Week 5
TOTAL BODY					
One-arm power snatch TB	5 × 2	5 × 4	5 × 2	5 × 4	5 × 2
Weight lifted					
One-arm split alt-foot snatch TB	5 × 2	5 × 4	5 × 2	5 × 4	5 × 2
Weight lifted					
LOWER BODY					
One-arm incline press CL	4 × 4	4 × 2	4 × 4	4 × 2	4 × 4
Weight lifted					
TRUNK					
Decline press crunch	3 × 12	3 × 12	3 × 12	3 × 12	3 × 12
Weight lifted					
Back extension	3 × 8	3 × 8	3 × 8	3 × 8	3 × 8
Weight lifted					
SHOULDERS					
Alt shoulder press CL	4 × 4	4 × 2	4 × 4	4 × 2	4 × 4
Weight lifted					

(continued)

Strength Cycle for Wrestlers *(continued)*

Thursday

Length 5 weeks

Goal Increase strength to improve balance and agility.

Intensity Complete the full number of required repetitions on the first set only. Use good form.

Pace Perform total-body lifts explosively. On all other exercises lift explosively and lower in 2 seconds.

Rest Take 2:30 between total-body exercises and 2:00 between all other sets and exercises.

Sets and Reps

Week	Strength cycle
1	TB = 5 × 2 CL = 4 × 2
2	TB = 5 × 4 CL = 4 × 4
3	TB = 5 × 2 CL = 4 × 2
4	TB = 5 × 4 CL = 4 × 4
5	TB = 5 × 2 CL = 4 × 2

	Week 1	Week 2	Week 3	Week 4	Week 5
TOTAL BODY					
One-arm power clean TB	5 × 2	5 × 4	5 × 2	5 × 4	5 × 2
Weight lifted					
Alt clean TB	5 × 2	5 × 4	5 × 2	5 × 4	5 × 2
Weight lifted					
LOWER BODY					
One-leg front squat CL	4 × 4	4 × 2	4 × 4	4 × 2	4 × 4
Weight lifted					
Side lunge CL	4 × 4	4 × 2	4 × 4	4 × 2	4 × 4
Weight lifted					
TRUNK					
Twisting crunch	3 × 12	3 × 12	3 × 12	3 × 12	3 × 12
Weight lifted					
BICEPS					
Alt reverse curl	3 × 5	3 × 5	3 × 5	3 × 5	3 × 5
Weight lifted					

Friday

Length 5 weeks

Goal Increase strength to improve balance and agility.

Intensity Complete the full number of required repetitions on the first set only. Use good form.

Pace Perform total-body lifts explosively. On all other exercises lift explosively and lower in 2 seconds.

Rest Take 2:30 between total-body exercises and 2:00 between all other sets and exercises.

Sets and Reps

Week	Strength cycle
1	TB = 5 × 2 CL = 4 × 2
2	TB = 5 × 4 CL = 4 × 4
3	TB = 5 × 2 CL = 4 × 2
4	TB = 5 × 4 CL = 4 × 4
5	TB = 5 × 2 CL = 4 × 2

	Week 1	Week 2	Week 3	Week 4	Week 5
TOTAL BODY					
One-arm power snatch TB	5 × 2	5 × 4	5 × 2	5 × 4	5 × 2
Weight lifted					
One-arm split alt-foot snatch TB	5 × 2	5 × 4	5 × 2	5 × 4	5 × 2
Weight lifted					
CHEST					
One-arm incline press CL	4 × 4	4 × 2	4 × 4	4 × 2	4 × 4
Weight lifted					
TRUNK					
V-up	3 × 12	3 × 12	3 × 12	3 × 12	3 × 12
Weight lifted					
Twisting back extension	3 × 8	3 × 8	3 × 8	3 × 8	3 × 8
Weight lifted					
SHOULDERS					
One-arm shoulder press CL	4 × 4	4 × 2	4 × 4	4 × 2	4 × 4
Weight lifted					

Strength Cycle for Soccer Players

Monday

Length 5 weeks

Goal Increase strength to improve balance and agility.

Intensity Complete the full number of required repetitions on each set.

Pace Perform total-body lifts explosively. On all other exercises lift as explosively as possible and lower in 2 seconds.

Rest Take 2:00 between all sets and exercises.

Sets and Reps

Week	Field players	Goalies
1	TB = 3 × 3 CL = 3 × 5	TB = 3 × 3 CL = 3 × 4
2	TB = 3 × 5 CL = 3 × 8	TB = 3 × 4 CL = 3 × 6
3	TB = 3 × 3 CL = 3 × 5	TB = 3 × 3 CL = 3 × 4
4	TB = 3 × 5 CL = 3 × 8	TB = 3 × 4 CL = 3 × 6
5	TB = 3 × 3 CL = 3 × 5	TB = 3 × 3 CL = 3 × 4

	Week 1	Week 2	Week 3	Week 4	Week 5
TOTAL BODY					
Split alt-foot alt jerk TB	3 × 3 + 3 × 3	3 × 5 + 3 × 4	3 × 3 + 3 × 3	3 × 5 + 3 × 4	3 × 3 + 3 × 3
Weight lifted					
LOWER BODY					
One-leg front squat CL	3 × 5 + 3 × 4	3 × 8 + 3 × 6	3 × 5 + 3 × 4	3 × 8 + 3 × 6	3 × 5 + 3 × 4
Weight lifted					
Side lunge	3 × 5 + 3 × 4	3 × 8 + 3 × 6	3 × 5 + 3 × 4	3 × 8 + 3 × 6	3 × 5 + 3 × 4
Weight lifted (total)					
TRUNK					
Overhead crunch throw	4 × 15 + 4 × 12	4 × 15 + 4 × 12	4 × 15 + 4 × 12	4 × 15 + 4 × 12	4 × 15 + 4 × 12
Weight lifted					
UPPER BODY					
Alt incline press CL	3 × 5 + 3 × 4	3 × 8 + 3 × 6	3 × 5 + 3 × 4	3 × 8 + 3 × 6	3 × 5 + 3 × 4
Weight lifted					
NECK					
MR flexion	1 × 8	1 × 8	1 × 8	1 × 8	1 × 8
Reps completed					

Wednesday

Length   5 weeks

Goal   Increase strength to improve balance and agility.

Intensity   Complete the full number of required repetitions on each set.

Pace   Perform total-body lifts explosively. On all other exercises lift as explosively as possible and lower in 2 seconds.

Rest   Take 2:00 between all sets and exercises.

Sets and Reps

Week	Field players	Goalies
1	TB = 3 × 3 CL = 3 × 5	TB = 3 × 3 CL = 3 × 4
2	TB = 3 × 5 CL = 3 × 8	TB = 3 × 4 CL = 3 × 6
3	TB = 3 × 3 CL = 3 × 5	TB = 3 × 3 CL = 3 × 4
4	TB = 3 × 5 CL = 3 × 8	TB = 3 × 4 CL = 3 × 6
5	TB = 3 × 3 CL = 3 × 5	TB = 3 × 3 CL = 3 × 4

	Week 1	Week 2	Week 3	Week 4	Week 5
TOTAL BODY					
Hang clean TB	3 × 3 + 3 × 3	3 × 5 + 3 × 4	3 × 3 + 3 × 3	3 × 5 + 3 × 4	3 × 3 + 3 × 5
Weight lifted					
LOWER BODY					
One-leg squat CL	3 × 5 + 3 × 4	3 × 8 + 3 × 6	3 × 5 + 3 × 4	3 × 8 + 3 × 6	3 × 5 + 3 × 4
Weight lifted					
TRUNK					
Plate lift twist	3 × 15 + 3 × 12	3 × 15 + 3 × 12	3 × 15 + 3 × 12	3 × 15 + 3 × 12	3 × 15 + 3 × 12
Weight lifted					
One-leg straight-leg deadlift CL	3 × 5 + 3 × 4	3 × 8 + 3 × 6	3 × 5 + 3 × 4	3 × 8 + 3 × 6	3 × 5 + 3 × 4
Weight lifted					
UPPER BODY					
Alt bench press CL	3 × 5 + 3 × 4	3 × 8 + 3 × 6	3 × 5 + 3 × 4	3 × 8 + 3 × 6	3 × 5 + 3 × 4
Weight lifted					
Pullover CL	3 × 5 + 3 × 4	3 × 8 + 3 × 6	3 × 5 + 3 × 4	3 × 8 + 3 × 6	3 × 5 + 3 × 4
Weight lifted					
NECK					
MR lateral flexion	1 × 8	1 × 8	1 × 8	1 × 8	1 × 8
Reps completed					

Strength Cycle for Ice Hockey Players

Monday

Length 5 weeks

Goal Increase strength to improve balance and agility.

Intensity Complete the full number of required repetitions on the first set only before increasing resistance.

Pace Perform total-body lifts explosively. On all other exercises lift explosively and lower in 2 seconds.

Rest Rest 2:15 between total-body sets and exercises and 2:00 between all other sets and exercises.

Sets and Reps

Week	Strength cycle
1	TB = 5 × 2 CL = 4 × 2
2	TB = 5 × 5 CL = 4 × 5
3	TB = 5 × 2 CL = 4 × 2
4	TB = 5 × 5 CL = 4 × 5
5	TB = 5 × 2 CL = 4 × 2

	Week 1	Week 2	Week 3	Week 4	Week 5
TOTAL BODY					
Alt power clean TB	5 × 2	5 × 5	5 × 2	5 × 5	5 × 2
Weight lifted					
One-arm clean TB	5 × 2	5 × 5	5 × 2	5 × 5	5 × 2
Weight lifted					
LOWER BODY					
One-leg squat CL	4 × 2	4 × 5	4 × 2	4 × 5	4 × 2
Weight lifted					
Lateral squat CL	4 × 2	4 × 5	4 × 2	4 × 5	4 × 2
Weight lifted					
TRUNK					
Twisting crunch	3 × 12	3 × 12	3 × 12	3 × 12	3 × 12
Weight lifted					
Twisting back extension	3 × 10	3 × 10	3 × 10	3 × 10	3 × 10
Weight lifted					
UPPER BACK					
Row CL	4 × 2	4 × 5	4 × 2	4 × 5	4 × 2
Weight lifted					
NECK					
MR lateral flexion	2 × 8	2 × 8	2 × 8	2 × 8	2 × 8
Reps completed					

Wednesday

Length 5 weeks

Goal Increase strength to improve balance and agility.

Intensity Complete the full number of required repetitions on the first set only before increasing resistance.

Pace Perform total-body lifts explosively. On all other exercises lift explosively and lower in 2 seconds.

Rest Rest 2:15 between total-body sets and exercises and 2:00 between all other sets and exercises.

Sets and Reps

Week	Strength cycle
1	TB = 5 × 2 CL = 4 × 2
2	TB = 5 × 5 CL = 4 × 5
3	TB = 5 × 2 CL = 4 × 2
4	TB = 5 × 5 CL = 4 × 5
5	TB = 5 × 2 CL = 4 × 2

	Week 1	Week 2	Week 3	Week 4	Week 5
TOTAL BODY					
One-arm power snatch TB	5 × 2	5 × 5	5 × 2	5 × 5	5 × 2
Weight lifted					
Split alt-foot alt snatch TB	5 × 2	5 × 5	5 × 2	5 × 5	5 × 2
Weight lifted					
CHEST					
Alt incline press CL	4 × 2	4 × 5	4 × 2	4 × 5	4 × 2
Weight lifted					
TRUNK					
Alt toe touch	3 × 12	3 × 12	3 × 12	3 × 12	3 × 12
Weight lifted					
Press crunch	3 × 12	3 × 12	3 × 12	3 × 12	3 × 12
Weight lifted					
SHOULDERS					
One-arm shoulder press	4 × 2	4 × 5	4 × 2	4 × 5	4 × 2
Weight lifted					
Alt lateral raise	3 × 6	3 × 6	3 × 6	3 × 6	3 × 6
Weight lifted					
NECK					
MR flexion and extension	2 × 8	2 × 8	2 × 8	2 × 8	2 × 8
Reps completed					

(continued)

Strength Cycle for Ice Hockey Players *(continued)*

Friday

<u>Length</u> 5 weeks

<u>Goal</u> Increase strength to improve balance and agility.

<u>Intensity</u> Complete the full number of required repetitions on the first set only before increasing resistance.

<u>Pace</u> Perform total-body lifts explosively. On all other exercises lift explosively and lower in 2 seconds.

<u>Rest</u> Rest 2:15 between total-body sets and exercises and 2:00 between all other sets and exercises.

Sets and Reps

Week	Strength cycle
1	TB = 5 × 2 CL = 4 × 2
2	TB = 5 × 5 CL = 4 × 5
3	TB = 5 × 2 CL = 4 × 2
4	TB = 5 × 5 CL = 4 × 5
5	TB = 5 × 2 CL = 4 × 2

	Week 1	Week 2	Week 3	Week 4	Week 5
TOTAL BODY					
Alt power jerk TB	5 × 2	5 × 5	5 × 2	5 × 5	5 × 2
Weight lifted					
Split alt-foot alt jerk TB	5 × 2	5 × 5	5 × 2	5 × 5	5 × 2
Weight lifted					
LOWER BODY					
One-leg front squat CL	4 × 2	4 × 5	4 × 2	4 × 5	4 × 2
Weight lifted					
Lunge CL	4 × 2	4 × 5	4 × 2	4 × 5	4 × 2
Weight lifted					
TRUNK					
Press crunch	3 × 12	3 × 12	3 × 12	3 × 12	3 × 12
Weight lifted					
Twisting back extension	3 × 10	3 × 10	3 × 10	3 × 10	3 × 10
Weight lifted					
CHEST					
Alt bench press CL	4 × 2	4 × 5	4 × 2	4 × 5	4 × 2
Weight lifted					
UPPER BACK					
Row CL	4 × 2	4 × 5	4 × 2	4 × 5	4 × 2
Weight lifted					

Strength Cycle for Downhill Skiers

Monday

Length 5 weeks

Goal Increase strength to improve balance and agility.

Intensity Complete the full number of required repetitions on the first set only before increasing resistance.

Pace Perform total-body lifts explosively. On all other exercises lift explosively and lower in 2 seconds.

Rest Rest 2:00 between total-body sets and exercises and 1:30 between all other sets and exercises.

Sets and Reps

Week	Strength cycle
1	TB = 5 × 3 CL = 4 × 4
2	TB = 5 × 5 CL = 4 × 6
3	TB = 5 × 3 CL = 4 × 4
4	TB = 5 × 5 CL = 4 × 6
5	TB = 5 × 3 CL = 4 × 4

	Week 1	Week 2	Week 3	Week 4	Week 5
TOTAL BODY					
One-arm power clean TB	5 × 3	5 × 5	5 × 3	5 × 5	5 × 3
Weight lifted					
Alt clean TB	5 × 3	5 × 5	5 × 3	5 × 5	5 × 3
Weight lifted					
LOWER BODY					
One-leg squat CL	4 × 4	4 × 6	4 × 4	4 × 6	4 × 4
Weight lifted					
Side lunge CL	4 × 4	4 × 6	4 × 4	4 × 6	4 × 4
Weight lifted					
TRUNK					
V-up	3 × 12	3 × 12	3 × 12	3 × 12	3 × 12
Weight lifted					
Twisting back extension	3 × 10	3 × 10	3 × 10	3 × 10	3 × 10
Weight lifted					
UPPER BACK					
Upright row CL	4 × 4	4 × 6	4 × 4	4 × 6	4 × 4
Weight lifted					

(continued)

Strength Cycle for Downhill Skiers *(continued)*

Wednesday

<u>Length</u> 5 weeks

<u>Goal</u> Increase strength to improve balance and agility.

<u>Intensity</u> Complete the full number of required repetitions on the first set only before increasing resistance.

<u>Pace</u> Perform total-body lifts explosively. On all other exercises lift explosively and lower in 2 seconds.

<u>Rest</u> Rest 2:00 between total-body sets and exercises and 1:30 between all other sets and exercises.

Sets and Reps

Week	Strength cycle
1	TB = 5 × 3 CL = 4 × 4
2	TB = 5 × 5 CL = 4 × 6
3	TB = 5 × 3 CL = 4 × 4
4	TB = 5 × 5 CL = 4 × 6
5	TB = 5 × 3 CL = 4 × 4

	Week 1	Week 2	Week 3	Week 4	Week 5
TOTAL BODY					
One-arm power jerk TB	5 × 3	5 × 5	5 × 3	5 × 5	5 × 3
Weight lifted					
Split alt-foot alt jerk TB	5 × 3	5 × 5	5 × 3	5 × 5	5 × 3
Weight lifted					
UPPER BODY					
One-arm bench press CL	4 × 6	4 × 4	4 × 6	4 × 4	4 × 6
Weight lifted					
TRUNK					
Decline twisting crunch	3 × 15	3 × 15	3 × 15	3 × 15	3 × 15
Weight lifted					
Back extension	3 × 12	3 × 12	3 × 12	3 × 12	3 × 12
Weight lifted					
TRICEPS					
Triceps extension AL	3 × 8	3 × 8	3 × 8	3 × 8	3 × 8
Weight lifted					

Friday

Length 5 weeks

Goal Increase strength to improve balance and agility.

Intensity Complete the full number of required repetitions on the first set only before increasing resistance.

Pace Perform total-body lifts explosively. On all other exercises lift explosively and lower in 2 seconds.

Rest Rest 2:00 between total-body sets and exercises and 1:30 between all other sets and exercises.

Sets and Reps

Week	Strength cycle
1	TB = 5 × 3 CL = 4 × 4
2	TB = 5 × 5 CL = 4 × 6
3	TB = 5 × 3 CL = 4 × 4
4	TB = 5 × 5 CL = 4 × 6
5	TB = 5 × 3 CL = 4 × 4

	Week 1	Week 2	Week 3	Week 4	Week 5
TOTAL BODY					
One-arm power snatch TB	5 × 3	5 × 5	5 × 3	5 × 5	5 × 3
Weight lifted					
Split alt-foot alt snatch TB	5 × 3	5 × 5	5 × 3	5 × 5	5 × 3
Weight lifted					
LOWER BODY					
Lunge CL	4 × 4	4 × 6	4 × 4	4 × 6	4 × 4
Weight lifted					
Straight-leg deadlift CL	4 × 4	4 × 6	4 × 4	4 × 6	4 × 4
Weight lifted					
TRUNK					
Press crunch	3 × 15	3 × 15	3 × 15	3 × 15	3 × 15
Weight lifted					
Back extension	3 × 12	3 × 12	3 × 12	3 × 12	3 × 12
Weight lifted					
UPPER BODY					
Incline press CL	4 × 4	4 × 6	4 × 4	4 × 6	4 × 4
Weight lifted					
Row CL	4 × 4	4 × 6	4 × 4	4 × 6	4 × 4
Weight lifted					

References

Introduction

Todd, J. 2003. The Strength Builders: A History of Barbells, Dumbbells and Indian Clubs. *The International Journal of the History of Sport.* 20(1): 65-90.

Chapter 1

Behm, D.G., E.J. Drinkwater, J.M. Willardson, M. Jeffrey, and P.M. Cowley. The role of instability rehabilitative resistance training for the core musculature. *Journal of Strength and Conditioning Research.* 33(3): 72-81.

Koshida, S., Y. Urabe, K. Miyashita, K. Iwai, and A. Kagimori. 2008. Muscular outputs during dynamic bench press under stable versus unstable conditions. *Journal of Strength and Conditioning Research.* 22(5): 1584-1588.

Lauder, M.A., and J.P. Lake. 2008. Biomechanical comparison of unilateral and bilateral power snatch lifts. *Journal of Strength and Conditioning Research.* 22(3): 653-660.

Welsch, E.A., M. Bird, J.L. Mayhew. 2005. Electromyography activity of the pectoralis major and anterior deltoid muscles during three upper body lifts. *Journal of Strength and Conditioning Research.* 19(2): 449-452.

Chapter 2

Wang, J. Physiological overview of conditioning training for college soccer athletes. *Strength Conditioning.* 17:62–65. 1995.

About the Author

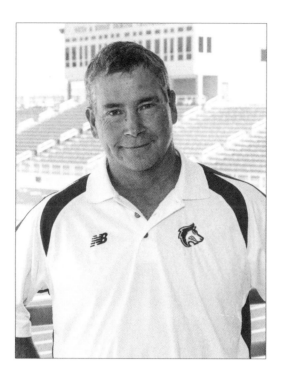

Allen Hedrick, MA, CSCS, RSCC, FNSCA, is the head strength and conditioning coach at Colorado State University at Pueblo, a position he has held since 2009. Hedrick began his coaching career as a graduate assistant strength and conditioning coach at Fresno State University. After graduation, Hedrick was hired at the Olympic Training Center in Colorado Springs as the strength and conditioning coordinator, a position he held for three years. Hedrick then moved on to the United States Air Force Academy, where he stayed for 12 years, the first three as an assistant and the final nine as the head strength and conditioning coach. Upon leaving the academy, Hedrick worked at the National Strength and Conditioning Association for three years, both in the Human Performance Center and in education, before moving to his current position. Hedrick, who was the NSCA's Collegiate Strength and Conditioning Coach of the Year in 2003, is a frequent publisher in various journals, has authored chapters in two text books, authored a book on strength and conditioning for football, produced numerous DVDs on a variety of strength and conditioning topics, and is a frequent speaker at conferences and clinics, both nationally and internationally.

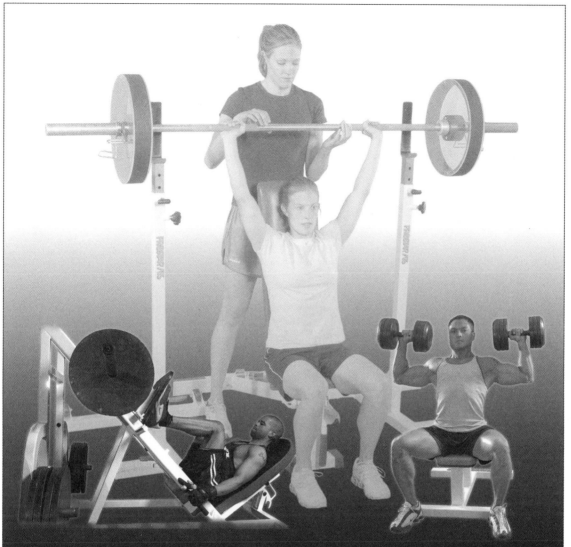

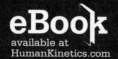